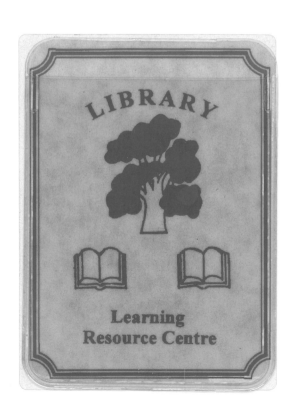

Next Generation Antidepressants

Moving Beyond Monoamines to Discover Novel Treatment Strategies for Mood Disorders

Next Generation Antidepressants

Moving Beyond Monoamines to Discover Novel Treatment Strategies for Mood Disorders

Edited by

Chad E. Beyer
Department of Pharmacology, University of Colorado School of Medicine Aurora, CO, USA

and

Stephen M. Stahl
Department of Psychiatry, University of California San Diego and Neuroscience Education Institute California, USA

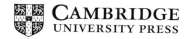
CAMBRIDGE
UNIVERSITY PRESS

CAMBRIDGE UNIVERSITY PRESS
Cambridge, New York, Melbourne, Madrid, Cape Town, Singapore,
São Paulo, Delhi, Dubai, Tokyo

Cambridge University Press
The Edinburgh Building, Cambridge CB2 8RU, UK

Published in the United States of America by Cambridge University Press, New York

www.cambridge.org
Information on this title: www.cambridge.org/9780521760584

© Cambridge University Press 2010

First published 2010

Printed in the United Kingdom at the University Press, Cambridge

A catalog record for this publication is available from the British Library

ISBN 978-0-521-76058-4 Hardback

Contents

Contributors

Lisa H. Berghorst, MA
Department of Psychology, Harvard
University, Cambridge, MA, USA

Chad E. Beyer, PhD, MBA
Department of Pharmacology, University of
Colorado School of Medicine, Aurora, CO,
USA

Adam M. Brickman, PhD
The Taub Institute for Research on
Alzheimer's Disease and the Aging Brain,
Columbia University, New York, NY, USA

Chun-Yu Chen, MS
Division of Mental Health and Addiction
Medicine, National Health Research
Institutes (NHRI), Taipei, Taiwan

Thomas I. F. H. Cremers, PhD
Brains On-Line BV, The Netherlands, and
Brains On-Line LLC, San Francisco, CA

Mark Day, PhD
Experimental Neuroimaging, Abbott
Laboratories, Abbott Park, IL, USA

Eliyahu Dremencov, PhD
Brains On-Line BV, Groningen, The
Netherlands

Malgorzata Filip, PhD, DSc
Laboratory of Drug Addiction Pharmacology,
Department of Pharmacology, Institute of
Pharmacology, Polish Academy of Sciences,
Krakow, Poland

Chris D. Griesemer, BS
The Center for Molecular and Genomic
Imaging, University of California, Davis,
CA, USA

Lotte de Groote, PhD
Solvay Pharmaceuticals Research
Laboratories, Weesp, The Netherlands

Keh-Ming Lin, MD, MPH
Center for Advanced Study in the
Behavioral Science, Stanford, California,
USA, and Division of Mental Health
and Addiction Medicine, National
Health Research Institutes (NHRI),
Taipei, Taiwan

Andrew C. McCreary, PhD
Solvay Pharmaceuticals Research
Laboratories, Weesp, The Netherlands

Laurence Mignon, PhD
Neuroscience Education Institute, Carlsbad,
CA, USA

Anna Parachikova, PhD
Cognitive Neuroscience, PsychoGenics, Inc,
Tarrytown, NY, USA

Roy H. Perlis, MD, MSc
Laboratory of Psychiatric
Pharmacogenomics, Center for Human
Genetic Research, Massachusetts General
Hospital, Boston, MA, USA

Diego A. Pizzagalli, PhD
Department of Psychology, Harvard
University, Cambridge, MA, USA

David P. Rotella, PhD
Chemical & Screening Sciences, Wyeth
Research, Princeton, NJ, USA

Jul Lea Shamy, PhD
Drug Discovery and Development,
PsychoGenics, Inc, Tarrytown, NY, USA

Stephen M. Stahl, MD, PhD
Department of Psychiatry, University
of California San Diego and
Neuroscience Education Institute,
Carlsbad, CA, USA

Yu-Jui Yvonne Wan, PhD
Department of Pharmacology,
Toxicology & Therapeutics, University
of Kansas Medical Center, Kansas City,
Kansas, USA

Preface

As the World Health Organization estimates that depression will become the second leading cause of death by the year 2020 – due primarily to complications arising from stress and the cardiovascular system – the need to develop novel and more effective treatment strategies for patients suffering with mood disorders has never been more paramount. Current treatment options for depressed patients include a variety of molecules designed to exclusively elevate central nervous system levels of monoamines such as serotonin (5-HT). These classes include the monoamine oxidase inhibitors and tricyclics and are exemplified by the selective serotonin reuptake inhibitors (SSRIs) and the dual serotonin/norepinephrine reuptake inhibitors (SNRIs). While these medicines are moderately effective in some patient populations, there are still considerable limitations associated with all commercially available antidepressants. These drawbacks include, but are not limited to, delayed onset of efficacy, treatment resistance in many patients, and deleterious side effects such as emesis and sexual dysfunction. The focus of this book is to review the current landscape and state of the field for depression research with an eye towards shedding light on where the future of mood disorders research is headed in terms of novel therapeutic targets, preclinical model development, exploring depression endophenotypes, and medicinal chemistry strategies. Undoubtedly all of these disciplines, as well as others including genetics and translational medicine approaches, will need to successfully collaborate to help build a better understanding of disease etiology, patient stratification, and treatment. As depression research has evolved over the past 50 years, the next decade will be instrumental in facilitating a move beyond our current understanding and pharmacological treatment options, and strive to discover and develop more personalized and effective treatment options for the millions of patients suffering from chronic and debilitating mood disorders.

Chad E. Beyer, PhD, MBA
Department of Pharmacology, University of Colorado School of Medicine, Aurora, CO, USA

Abbreviations

5HIAA, 5-hydroxy-indole-acetic acid
ACTH, adrenocorticotropic hormone
BBB, blood–brain barrier
BD, bipolar disorder
BDI, Beck Depression Inventory
BDNF, brain-derived neurotrophic factor
BNST, bed nucleus of the stria terminalis
BOLD, blood oxygen level-dependent
CANTAB, Cambridge Neuropsychological Test Automated Battery
CBF, cerebral blood flow
CBV, cerebral blood volume
CNV, copy-number variation
CRF, corticotropin-releasing factor
CSF, cerebrospinal fluid
DA, dopamine
DAT, dopamine transporter
DRN, dorsal raphe nucleus
DST, dexamethasone suppression test
ECT, electro-convulsive therapy
ERP, event-related potential
FDG, fluorine-18-labeled deoxyglucose
FLAIR, fluid attenuated inverse recovery
fMRI, functional magnetic resonance imaging
FST, forced swim test
GWAS, genomewide association study
HPA, hypothalamic–pituitary–adrenal
IAT, Implicit Association Test
LC, locus coeruleus
MAOI, monoamine oxidase inhibitor
MDD, major depressive disorder
MED, minimal effective dose
MTD, maximal tolerated dose
MRN, median raphe nucleus
MRS, magnetic resonance spectroscopy
MTHF, L-5-methyl-tetrahydrofolate
NE, norepinephrine
NET, norepinephrine transporter
NK, neurokinin
PET, positron emission tomography
PFC, prefrontal cortex
phMRI, pharmacological MRI
POC, proof-of-concept

SERT, serotonin transporter
SNP, single nucleotide polymorphism
SNRI, serotonin/norepinephrine reuptake inhibitor
SP, substance P
SSRI, selective serotonin reuptake inhibitor
STAR*D, Sequenced Treatment Alternatives to Relieve Depression study
SXR, steroid and xenobiotic receptor
T3, triiodothyronine
TCA, tricyclic antidepressant
TCI, Temperament and Character Inventory
TST, tail suspension test
vACC, ventral anterior cingulate cortex
VTA, ventral tegmental area
WCST, Wisconsin Card Sorting Test
WGTA, Wisconsin General Testing Apparatus
WMH, white matter hyperintensities

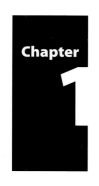

Chapter

1

Current depression landscape: a state of the field today

Laurence Mignon and Stephen M. Stahl

Abstract

More than two dozen pharmacological treatments are currently available for depression, working by more than a half dozen mechanisms, yet there remain many unmet therapeutic needs. Available antidepressants act directly on monoamine mechanisms, influencing receptors and transporters for serotonin, norepinephrine, and/or dopamine. Truly novel therapeutic targets beyond the monoamines have not emerged in the past few decades. Advances have been mostly in improved tolerability, and as a result, limitations in efficacy persist for all agents in the antidepressant class. Specifically, far too few patients, perhaps only a third, attain a full remission of symptoms, and those who have had many episodes of depression are not likely to sustain any remission for more than a few months. Thus, there is the urgent need for antidepressants with improved efficacy. Although the "holy grail" of antidepressant treatment has long been rapid onset of action, the reality is that more robust and sustained efficacy, even if delayed, is the unmet need of today. This is unlikely to be met by targeting the same monoamine transporters and receptors where current antidepressants act, so novel therapeutic targets must be identified if there is to be novel therapeutic efficacy of more robust and sustained antidepressant action.

Other issues in the treatment of depression include the increasing confusion between unipolar and bipolar depression, particularly at onset of first depressive episodes, as well as the confusion between treatment-resistant unipolar depression versus difficult-to-treat rapid cycling, mixed episodes of bipolar depression. Treatments for bipolar depression such as anticonvulsants and atypical antipsychotics are increasingly being used for bipolar and treatment-resistant cases. Future therapeutics may usefully exploit these mechanisms, and treatment of difficult cases in the future will likely involve use of multiple simultaneous mechanisms, either with multiple drugs or with multifunctional drugs.

There is also concern that depression may be a progressive illness, with unipolar depression progressing to treatment-resistant depression or even to bipolar spectrum disorder, and bipolar disorder progressing to rapid cycling and mixed treatment-resistant bipolar episodes. Future treatments of depression may not only have the potential to treat current symptoms and prevent their relapse, but also to halt progression and thus be disease-modifying, altering the course of untreated or inadequately treated illness.

At the beginning there were three monoamines . . .

The World Health Organization estimates that depression is the fourth leading cause of disability worldwide, with a lifetime prevalence of about 15–20% [1]. The first reports of antidepressant treatments date back to the early 1950s, when researchers in the United States

Next Generation Antidepressants: Moving Beyond Monoamines to Discover Novel Treatment Strategies for Mood Disorders, ed. Chad E. Beyer and Stephen M. Stahl. Published by Cambridge University Press.
© Cambridge University Press 2010.

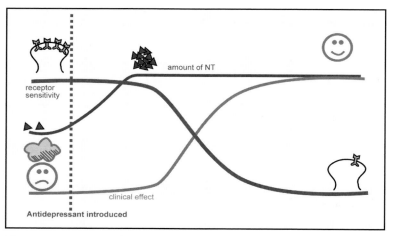

Figure 1.1 Time course of antidepressant effects. Depicted here is the time course for (1) clinical changes, (2) neurotransmitter changes, and (3) receptor sensitivity changes following antidepressant treatment. The amount of neurotransmitter changes rapidly following the introduction of an antidepressant. The clinical effect, however, is delayed, as is the downregulation of neurotransmitter receptors. The temporal correlation between the changes in clinical effect and the changes in receptor sensitivity has prompted researchers to posit the hypothesis that changes in neurotransmitter receptor sensitivity may actually induce the clinical effects of antidepressant medications. Besides the antidepressant and anxiolytic actions, these clinical effects also include tolerance to the acute side effects of these medications.

and in Europe simultaneously reported that two antituberculosis agents, isonazid and iproniazid, had mood-enhancing properties in patients [2,3]. It was not until the late 1950s that an opportune discovery of mood-enhancing effects of tricyclic (three rings) drugs led to the first antidepressant. Unfortunately, at the time, the number of people diagnosed with depression who would benefit from these "new" drugs remained low (50–100 per million), so this was not the top priority of the pharmaceutical companies [4]. The big blockbuster drug for depression only hit the market in 1988, when the Food and Drug Administration approved the first selective serotonin reuptake inhibitor (SSRI), fluoxetine. This "legitimized" depression as an important disorder for the pharmaceutical industry to investigate and develop better pharmacotherapies for.

Based on the monoamine hypothesis of depression, which posits a lack in monoamines in various brain regions of depressed patients, the development of antidepressant medications has focused on increasing the levels and synaptic effects of three monoamines: the catecholamines dopamine and norepinephrine, and the indoleamine serotonin [5]. The mechanism of action by which an increase in monoamines is generated often includes blockade of the various transporters for these monoamines, namely the dopamine transporter (DAT), the norepinephrine transporter (NET), and the serotonin transporter (SERT). However, the monoamine levels can increase quite rapidly following blockade of these transporters, while the clinical benefits of antidepressants often lag behind this effect by weeks. The neurotransmitter receptor sensitivity hypothesis of depression can explain this lag time, and is in line with the neurotransmitter receptor hypothesis that focuses on the abnormal upregulation of receptors in depression. By elevating neurotransmitter levels for an extended period of time, antidepressants can lead to the downregulation of the pathologic receptor upregulation. This is consistent with the time required to obtain clinical efficacy upon initiation of antidepressant treatment (Figure 1.1).

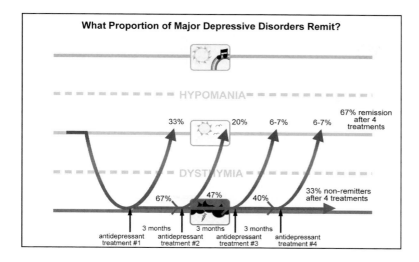

Figure 1.2
Remission rates in major depressive disorder. It has been estimated that one-third of patients with depression will remit during the first treatment with any antidepressant. For those who do not remit, the likelihood of remission with another antidepressant monotherapy decreases with each additional trial. After four sequential 12-week treatments only two-thirds of patients will have achieved full remission.

Of course, the changes in receptor number or sensitivity obtained following antidepressant effects certainly also require alterations in gene expression, transcription, and translation, and in the production of various neurotrophic factors. Preclinical studies have shown that brain-derived neurotrophic factor (BDNF) is one candidate whose expression levels are increased following antidepressant treatment [6]. Thus, besides modulating monoamine and receptor levels, the final common pathway to all antidepressants may be the regulation of various trophic factors.

STAR*D and treatment approaches

While many patients respond favorably to the antidepressants currently on the market, a significant number experience residual symptoms, treatment resistance, and relapse. The recent STAR*D (Sequenced Treatment Alternatives to Relieve Depression) study [7] has shed some light on the reality of antidepressant treatment. Initially, only one-third of patients on citalopram monotherapy remitted. The other two-thirds who failed to remit saw their likelihood of remission decrease with each successive trial of another antidepressant mono-therapy. Thus, after 4 successive monotherapies were tried for 12 weeks each, i.e. after one year of treatment, only two-thirds of patients achieved remission (Figure 1.2). Additionally, the more treatment cycles it took to get the patient to remit, the higher the likelihood of relapse.

The STAR*D results has sent a shockwave through the medical community, as it debunked previously held beliefs that major depressive disorder was highly treatable, and that some antidepressants were superior in efficacy to others. The results have also high-lighted the need to further explore more effective treatment methods for major depressive disorder. New treatments are currently under development or have just hit the market, and these include new formulations of old antidepressants, new medications focusing on the monoamine hypothesis of depression, and experimental agents with novel mechanisms of action (see the section on improving treatments).

If multiple successive monotherapies with one antidepressant are not the way to effec-tively treat major depressive disorder, then what actions should be implemented to ascertain

Table 1.1 Stages of primary unipolar depression (adapted from [13]).

1.	Prodromal phase (anxiety, irritable mood, anhedonia, sleep disorders)
	a. no depressive symptoms
	b. minor depression
2.	Major depressive episode
3.	Residual phase
	a. no depressive symptoms
	b. dysthymia
4.	a. recurrent depression
	b. double depression
5.	Chronic major depressive episode (lasting at least 2 years without interruptions)

maximum benefit to the patient? Some experts are suggesting that it may be beneficial to use augmentation and combination strategies from the outset of the first treatment in order to enhance the outcome of the treatment, namely remission. The synergistic effect of multiple medications combined with their broader spectrum of action may prevent the initiation of oppositional tolerance [8,9]. However, besides developing better pharmacological treatment approaches, the field of psychiatry may also want to borrow from general medicine, and adopt the "staging method" to properly diagnose the big picture of depression [10,11]. While the DSM-IV looks at depression as a flat, cross-sectional view of the patient's ailments, the "staging method" takes into account the longitudinal development of depression, including previous episodes and the response to previous treatments. Primary unipolar depression, for example, has been divided into five stages: a prodromal phase can lead to the major depressive episode which can result in a residual phase that can escalate into recurrent depression and finally chronic depressive episodes (see Table 1.1) [12].

While this type of staging of major depression may already occur behind a psychiatrist's door, its application may need to be expanded to all healthcare practitioners, as it could impact on the success of a pharmacological treatment as well. A medication that may be useful in one stage may be less efficacious in another; or psychosocial therapy in conjunction with pharmacotherapy may be more beneficial in severe versus chronic depression [13]. Thus it becomes important to adopt a holistic view when talking about diagnosis and treatment of major depressive disorder.

Improving treatments: "make-over" of old medications

In order to improve tolerability and thus adherence to medications, it may be necessary to further investigate different formulations of old medications. Recently, bupropion has been developed in a hydrobromide salt formulation instead of the traditional hydrochloride salt formulation. This allows for higher doses (mg equivalency to buproprion hydrochloride salt) to be packaged into one pill, therefore potentially facilitating higher dosing in treatment-resistant patients.

Trazodone is currently undergoing a "make over" and waiting for approval of its new high-dose (300–450 mg), once-daily controlled release formulation. This formulation would allow patients to take the necessary higher doses without experiencing the sedatory side effects the following day.

The active metabolite of venlaflaxine, desvenlaflaxine, is being "made over" into its own legitimate antidepressant. Being produced following enzymatic activity by CYP450 2D6, desvenlaflaxine is less metabolized than the mother compound and may thus allow for more stable plasma levels [14]. Like venlaflaxine, desvenlaflaxine is a more potent inhibitor of SERT than NET, but when compared to the same doses of venlaflaxine, desvenlaflaxine exhibits greater potency at NET than SERT. This property may render it a perfect candidate to treat painful and vasomotor symptoms, which are theoretically due to a malfunctioning NE system. Desvenlaflaxine is also efficacious at treating hot flushes associated with perimenopause, but due to cardiovascular safety concerns is not approved for such use [5,15].

Improving treatments: new ways to tweak monoamine levels

Atypical antipsychotics exhibit different degrees of success when treating the depressed phase of bipolar disorder [5]. This is most likely the result of their very elaborate receptor profile, as they can lead to increased levels of serotonin, norepinephrine, and dopamine, either directly or indirectly. Their mood-enhancing property can result from the direct blockade of NET thus increasing norepinephrine levels, or the direct blockade of SERT thus increasing serotonin levels. Indirect action via the alpha 2 receptors can lead to enhanced norepinephrine and serotonin levels, and modulation of various serotonin receptors including the 5HT2A, 5HT2C, and 5HT1A can, by disinhibiting norepinephrine and dopamine, indirectly result in increased levels of these monoamines.

As atypical antipsychotics are an eclectic mix of different compounds, they also treat the depressed phase of bipolar disorder with varying efficacy in different patients. Quetiapine appears to have the highest efficacy as monotherapy in the treatment of bipolar depression. At the correct doses, its active metabolite norquetiapine leads to just the appropriate mix of receptor modulation, namely less than full saturation of D2 receptors, proper inhibition of 5HT2C receptors and NET, and adequate stimulation of 5HT1A receptors [5,14]. One limitation as to whether these compounds will become mainstream in the treatment of unipolar depression may depend on their side effect and cost profile [16].

The search for the most efficacious antidepressant first took pharmacologists down the road of finding the most selective compound, such as the SSRI. Then pharmacologists developed compounds that selectively blocked two monoamines, for example serotonin and norepinephrine reuptake inhibitors. Today, the idea that a triple reuptake inhibitor may be the answer is gaining momentum. Table 1.2 lists different triple reuptake inhibitors, which target the serotonin, dopamine, and norepinephrine transporter with varying degrees. Full blockade of all three monoamine transporters is not optimal, and these compounds are trying to find the best balance that will lead to the most efficacious monoaminergic activity.

Another new group of compounds which have gained interest in the treatment of depression are the norepinephrine dopamine disinhibitors, or, simply stated, agents that block the 5HT2C receptors. The new antidepressant agomelatine, for example, is a potent 5HT2C blocker in addition to being an agonist at the melatonin 1 and 2 receptors; thus besides treating the symptoms of depression, it may be beneficial in improving sleep issues [14]. Table 1.3 lists the new agents in development that are targeting the different serotonin receptors.

Table 1.2 Triple reuptake inhibitors currently in development as antidepressants (table adapted from [17]).

Triple reuptake inhibitor	Additional receptor properties	Stage of development
DOV 216303		Phase II depression
DOV 21947		Phase II depression
GW 372475 (NS2359)		No ongoing clinical trials in depression; Phase II for attention deficit hyperactivity disorder
Boehringer/ NS2330		No ongoing clinical trials in depression; Phase II for Alzheimer dementia and for Parkinson's disease discontinued
NS2360		Preclinical
Sepracor SEP 225289		Phase II depression
Lu AA24530	5HT2C, 5HT3, 5HT2A, alpha 1A	Phase II depression
Lu AA37096	5HT6	Phase I
Lu AA34893	5HT2A, alpha 1A, and 5HT6	Phase II depression

Table 1.3 Serotonergic agents currently in development as antidepressants (table adapted from [17]).

New serotonergic targets	Agent	Additional receptor properties	Stage of development
5HT2C antagonism	Agomelatine	Melatonin 1 and 2	Approved EMEA with liver monitoring, Phase III depression in USA
SSRI/5HT3 antagonism	Lu AA21004	5HT1A	Phase III depression
SSRI/5HT1A partial agonism	Vilazodone (SB 659746A)		Phase III depression
5HT1A partial agonism	Gepirone ER		Late-stage development for depression
5HT1A partial agonism	PRX 00023		Phase II depression
5HT1A partial agonism	MN 305		No clinical trials in depression; Phase II/III for generalized anxiety disorder
Sigma 1/5HT1A partial agonism	VPI 013 (OPC 14523)	Serotonin transporter	Phase II depression
5HT1A agonism/ 5HT2A antagonism	TGW-00-AD/ AA		Phase II depression
SRI/5HT2/5HT1A/ 5HT1D	TGBA-01-AD		Phase II depression
5HT1B/D antagonism	Elzasonan		Phase II depression

Improving treatments: looking beyond the monoamines

While modulation of the three monoamines has had great success in the treatment of depression, it may be necessary to go beyond the monoamines to find newer, more efficacious drugs or better augmenting agents for difficult-to-treat or treatment-resistant depression. The medical food L-5-methyl-tetrahydrofolate (MTHF), a key derivative of folate, is an important player in the synthesis of monoamines, and if delivered directly to the brain can theoretically increase the levels of all monoamines [5], especially in patients who have not responded to previous antidepressant medications and who have low folate levels [18].

Table 1.4 lists a large number of novel agents with new targets that are either in pre-clinical or early clinical development [5]. These agents range from low-molecular-weight compounds acting at the hypothalamic–pituitary–adrenal axis to neurokinin receptor antagonists.

Thus, the search for the next antidepressant is certainly an interesting one, and can either build on properties already known to work or on new ideas that just may give us the "silver bullet" we are looking for.

Unipolar versus bipolar depression: are these present along a progressive mood disorder spectrum?

A major impediment regarding the adequate treatment of unipolar disorder has been the fact that a large proportion of patients initially diagnosed with unipolar depression actually have bipolar II disorder (Figure 1.3). Patients with bipolar II disorder spend more time in the depressed state than either the (hypo)manic or mixed states, and can be easily misdiagnosed with unipolar depression if a proper history is not taken. This unfortunately results in them being treated first with an antidepressant – which could lead to activation and mood cycling, and worse to suicidality – instead of receiving the proper treatment of lithium, an anticonvulsant mood stabilizer, or an atypical antipsychotic.

Successful recognition of whether a depressed patient has a bipolar disorder or unipolar depression lies in obtaining the proper family and medical history, as the symptoms the patient will present with are similar in unipolar versus bipolar depression (Figure 1.4). Patterns of past symptoms and the response to prior antidepressants, as well as current symptoms such as more time sleeping, overeating, comorbid anxiety, motor retardation, mood liability, or psychotic or suicidal thoughts can all be used to correctly discriminate unipolar depression from bipolar depression [5].

It also remains to be determined whether continuity exists between bipolar disorder and major depressive disorder. A review of the scientific literature suggests that a categorical approach may be best applicable when discussing the extremes of the mood spectrum, such as bipolar I and major depressive disorder, while midway disorders such as bipolar II and major depressive disorder plus bipolar signs should best be seen along a continuum or a spectrum [19]. Thus it is not yet clear whether all mood disorders should be placed on a spectrum, and therefore whether they should be treated using the same approach.

Another question that remains unanswered thus far is whether mood disorders such as unipolar depression and bipolar disorders are progressive (Figure 1.5). If unipolar depression is untreated or undertreated, will the presence of residual symptoms or even relapses lead to a deterioration of the illness accompanied by more frequent recurrences, shorter inter-episode recoveries and even potentially treatment resistance? Additionally, could this

Table 1.4 New compounds currently in development as antidepressants (table adapted from [17]).

New mechanism	Agent	Stage of development
Beta 3 agonism	Amibegron	Phase III discontinued
Neurokinin (NK) 2 antagonism	Saredutant (SR48968)	Phase III discontinued
NK2 antagonism	SAR 1022279	Preclinical
NK2 antagonism	SSR 241586 (NK2 and NK3)	Preclinical
NK2 antagonism	SR 144190	Phase I
NK2 antagonism	GR 159897	Preclinical
NK3 antagonism	Osanetant (SR142801)	No current clinical trials in depression; preliminary trials in schizophrenia
NK3 antagonism	Talnetant (SB223412)	No current clinical trials in depression; Phase II for schizophrenia and for irritable bowel syndrome
NK3 antagonism	SR 146977	Preclinical
Substance P antagonism	Aprepitant [MK869; L-754030 (Emend)]	Phase III discontinued
Substance P antagonism	L-758,298; L-829,165; L-733,060	No clinical trials in depression; Phase III for nausea/ vomiting
Substance P antagonism	CP122721; CP99994; CP96345	Phase II depression
Substance P antagonism	Casopitant (GW679769)	No clinical trials in depression; Phase III for nausea/ vomiting
Substance P antagonism	Vestipitant (GW 597599) +/− paroxetine	No clinical trials in depression; Phase II for social anxiety disorder
Substance P antagonism	LY 686017	No clinical trials in depression; Phase II for social anxiety disorder and for alcohol dependence/ craving
Substance P antagonism	GW823296	Phase I
Substance P antagonism	(Nolpitantium) SR140333	No clinical trials in depression; Phase II for ulcerative colitis
Substance P antagonism	SSR240600; R-673	No clinical trials in depression; Phase II for overactive bladder
Substance P antagonism	NKP-608; AV608	No clinical trials in depression; Phase II for social anxiety disorder
Substance P antagonism	CGP49823	Preclinical
Substance P antagonism	SDZ NKT 34311	Preclinical
Substance P antagonism	SB679769	Preclinical
Substance P antagonism	GW597599	Phase II depression
Substance P antagonism	Vafopitant (GR205171)	No clinical trials in depression; Phase II for insomnia and for post-traumatic stress disorder
MIF-1 pentapeptide analog	Nemifitide (INN 00835)	Phase II depression – trial suspended
MIF-1 pentapeptide analog	5-Hydroxy-nemifitide (INN 01134)	Preclinical

Table 1.4 (cont.)

New mechanism	Agent	Stage of development
Glucocorticoid antagonism	Mifepristone (Corlux)	Phase III depression
Glucocorticoid antagonism	Org 34517; Org 34850 (glucocorticoid receptor II antagonists)	Phase III depression
corticotropin-releasing factor (CRF) 1 antagonism	R121919	Phase I
CRF1 antagonism	CP316,311	Phase II (trial terminated)
CRF1 antagonism	BMS 562086	Phase II
CRF1 antagonism	GW876008	No clinical trials in depression; Phase II for social anxiety disorder and for irritable bowel syndrome
CRF1 antagonism	ONO-233M	Preclinical
CRF1 antagonism	JNJ19567470; TS041	Preclinical
CRF1 antagonism	SSR125543	Phase I
CRF1 antagonism	SSR126374	Preclinical
Vasopressin 1B antagonism	SSR149415	Phase II

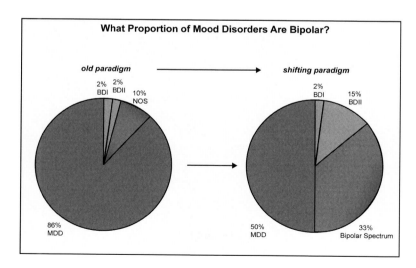

Figure 1.3 Incidence of mood disorders. Diagnoses of bipolar disorder (BD) have become increasingly common in recent years. Although many patients who would have previously been diagnosed with major depressive disorder (MOD) (old paradigm) are now being diagnosed with bipolar disorder (shifting paradigm), the syndrome can be hard to detect. There are still a large number of patients who go many years without an accurate diagnosis of bipolar disorder.

vicious circle of relapses lead to bipolar disorder? In the same line of thought, untreated or undertreated manic or depressive episodes could result in mixed and dysphoric episodes which could finally evolve into rapid cycling and treatment-resistant bipolar disorders. The balance between overdiagnosis and underdiagnosis of mood disorders is quite sensitive: is it

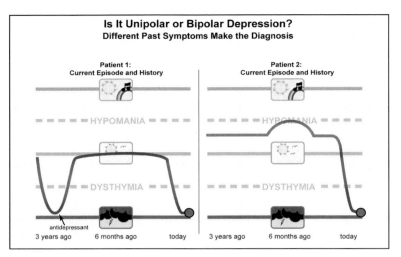

Figure 1.4 Unipolar versus bipolar depression. Both patients in this mood chart are "today" presenting with identical current symptoms of a major depressive episode (gray dot in the figure). Patient 1, however, has unipolar depression while patient 2 has bipolar depression. The pattern of past symptoms is relevant and can help distinguish between both disorders: patient 1 has experienced a prior depressive episode, while patient 2 has had a prior hypomanic episode. Gaining a complete picture may often require additional interviews with family members or close friends of the patient.

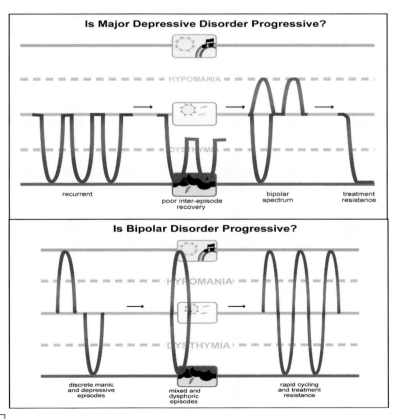

Figure 1.5 Are mood disorders progressive? (Top) It has been suggested that un(der)treated unipolar depression could develop into a bipolar spectrum condition, and could eventually reach the point of treatment resistance. (Bottom) It has further been posited that un(der) treated or mistreated episodes of mania and depression could develop into mixed or dysphoric episodes, rapid cycling and also finally into treatment resistance.

best to be less conservative in the hope that the diabolical learning of the brain pathways can be stopped and that prevention of these aberrant neuronal connections will reduce the risk of treatment-resistant disorders? The answer to this question is still being investigated.

Conclusion

The more we understand about the underlying neurobiology of depression and the effectiveness of current treatments, the closer we will get to individualizing patient care. By having a vast array of different treatment options, such as new formulations of old drugs, more selective compounds, as well as more elaborate combinations of triple reuptake inhibitors, clinicians will be able to customize their treatment approach and reach the ultimate goal in the treatment of depression, namely remission.

References

1. Rubinow, D. R. 2006. *N. Engl. J. Med.*, **354**, 1305.

2. Selikoff, I. J., and Robitzek, E. H. 1952. *Dis. Chest*, **21**(4), 385.

3. Healy, D. 1996. *The Psychopharmacologists: Interviews*, London, Chapman & Hall.

4. Healy, D. 1999. *J. Nerv. Ment. Dis.*, **187**(3), 174.

5. Stahl, S. M. 2008. *Stahl's Essential Psychopharmacology*, third edition, New York, Cambridge University Press.

6. Duman, R. S., Nakagawa, S., and Malberg, J. 2001. *Neuropsychopharmacology*, **25**, 836.

7. Warden, D., Rush, A. J., Trivedi, M. H., Fava, M., and Wisniewski, S. R. 2007. *Curr. Psychiatry. Rep.*, **9**, 449.

8. Fava, M., and Rush, A. J. 2006. *Psychother. Psychosom.*, **75**, 139.

9. Fava, G. A. 2003. *J. Clin. Psychiatry*, **64**, 123.

10. Fava, G. A., and Kellner, R. 1993. *Acta Psychiatr. Scand.*, **87**, 223.

11. McGorry, P. D., Hichie, I. B., Yang, A. R., Pantelis, C., and Jackson, H. J. 2006. *Aust. N. Z. J. Psychiatry*, **40**, 616.

12. Fava, G. A., and Tossani, E. 2007. *Early Interv. Psychiatry*, **1**, 9.

13. Fava, G. A., Tomba, E., and Grandi, S. 2007. *Psychother. Psychosom.*, **76**, 260.

14. Stahl, S. M. 2009. *Essential Psychopharmacology: The Prescriber's Guide*, third edition, New York, Cambridge University Press.

15. Wise, D. D., Felker, A., and Stahl, S. M. 2008. *CNS Spectr.*, **13**, 647.

16. Papakostas, G. I., Shelton, R. C., Smith, J., and Fava, M. 2007. *J. Clin. Psychiatry*, **68**, 826.

17. Grady, M. M., and Stahl, S. M. 2010. *Encyclopedia of Psychopharmacology*, Heidelberg, Springer-Verlag.

18. Fava, M. 2007. *J. Clin. Psychiatry*, **68**(suppl 10), 4.

19. Benazzi, F. 2007. *Psychother. Psychosom.*, **76**, 70.

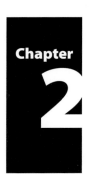

Novel therapeutic targets for treating affective disorders

Eliyahu Dremencov and Thomas I. F. H. Cremers

Abstract

Prevalence of depression has increased progressively over the last decades. Besides the impact on human quality of life, the pharmaco-economical impact of this syndrome requires ongoing development of newer, more powerful antidepressants. While optimizing existing therapeutic compounds, multiple approaches can be taken to generate superiority over these compounds. The delay in onset of action of antidepressants is of relevance as the presence of side effects during the initial absence of clinical effects causes low therapy compliance. Obviously, a decrease in onset of action would overcome this problem. Current therapy still induces considerable side effects depending on the class of antidepressants used. Reducing these has multiple advantages, such as it will increase compliance but also facilitate the rapid and safe initiation of drug treatment. In line with safety requirements is the notion that new antidepressants should not be prone to hazardous effects in overdose, nor should they induce dangerous interactions by interfering with other treatment. Finally, it is currently recognized that depression is a cluster of symptoms rather than a concise disease. To this end, it is recognized that more tailored treatments might be required in the future. Arguably targeting subsymptoms and comorbid features such as anxiety are of high relevance. Attempts to improve antidepressants have been made into monoamine-related strategies, but also more recently in non-monoamine strategies. The effectiveness of monoamine-targeted selective, dual- and triple-uptake inhibitors and augmented uptake inhibitors is discussed. In addition, new strategies such as monoamine non-uptake inhibitor drugs or non-monoamine drugs exerting effects on Glu, gamma-aminobutyric acid (GABA), Substance P, and acetylcholine are discussed, as are more miscellaneous approaches.

Major depression: overview

Depression is a syndrome that causes high morbidity and mortality. The illness is characterized by a high degree of heritability and affects about 20% of the population. The World Health Organization predicts that towards the year 2020, depression will become the second leading cause of death in the world.

Depression subtypes

Specialists commonly agree that depression is a syndrome rather than a single illness. The Hamilton depression rating scale (HAM-D scale) classifies multiple subtypes of depression.

Next Generation Antidepressants: Moving Beyond Monoamines to Discover Novel Treatment Strategies for Mood Disorders, ed. Chad E. Beyer and Stephen M. Stahl. Published by Cambridge University Press.
© Cambridge University Press 2010.

Besides major depression, subtypes are characterized by the abundance of psychotic features (bipolar and), or other miscellaneous features.

Comorbidity

Depression is present with high comorbidity of multiple other psychiatric features such as anxiety, cognitive perturbations, limited sleep quality and duration, and psychotic episodes. Given these variable perturbations in depressed patients, it is important to realize that depression should be treated as a syndrome with variable symptoms, rather than a confined illness with a specific treatment.

Clinical effectiveness; onset, short-term efficacy, prevention from relapse, comorbid targets

When studying the effectiveness of antidepressants, multiple issues have to be taken into consideration. On one side it should be realized that clinical effectiveness is generally estimated from short-term efficacy studies. Although it is of importance that the apparent lag time between onset of activity and start of treatment is as short as possible, this readout does not contain multiple other parameters which are of importance in overall drug treatment. Prevention against relapse illustrates the long-term benefits of treatment.

Monoamine theory of depression

Several decades ago it was discovered that monoamine oxidase inhibitors (MAOIs) were effective antidepressants. Soon after, tricyclic antidepressants (TCAs) were also found to be effective in this disorder, and since their pharmacological effects comprised monoamine reuptake inhibition, it was hypothesized that a deficiency in monoamines might be responsible for depression. This hypothesis as proposed by Schildkraut in 1965 [1] is known as the monoamine hypothesis of depression. Several studies have been performed evaluating the homeostasis of monoamines function in depressed patients.

5-Hydroxy-indole-acetic acid in cerebrospinal fluid (CSF)

Most investigators have observed decreased CSF levels of 5-HIAA in depressed patients when compared to normal controls. This observation was hypothesized to be related to decreased serotonin metabolism in the brain of depressed patients [2–6]. More recent studies, however, have been unable to observe similar relations, and found more evidence for low CSF 5-HIAA levels to be related to violence and suicide, rather than depression [7].

Post-mortem brain tissue

Reports on 5-HT levels measured in post-mortem brain tissue have been somewhat conflicting. Whereas most studies indicate that 5-HIAA levels (and hence metabolic breakdown) are lower in raphe nuclei of depressed patients [8,9], conflicting results exist on 5-HIAA and 5-HT content in other parts of the brain [10]. However, post-mortem artifacts and therapy-induced changes in content may have complicated the results.

Evidence from therapeutic interventions

The notion that LSD, a potent serotonin receptor antagonist, could induce mood changes in humans gave rise to the idea that serotonin could be involved in the etiology of mood disorders [1,11,12]. This idea was strengthened by the observation that reserpine, a mono-amine depleter, was able to induce depressive symptoms in humans [13]. The effectiveness of MAOIs and TCAs in the treatment of depression gave further support for a role of serotonin in depression.

These observations have initiated the development of multiple selective serotonin uptake inhibitors (SSRIs), which have been the treatment of choice for depression for the last decade.

Existing antidepressants: tricyclic antidepressants and selective serotonin reuptake inhibitors-efficacy and side-effect profiles

SSRIs and the serotonergic system

The serotonergic innervation of the brain mainly originates in the dorsal raphe nucleus (DRN) and the median raphe nucleus (MRN). These nuclei innervate a variety of structures within the brain, with a topical organization with respect to several brain areas. Whereas the prefrontal cortex (PFC) is mainly innervated by the DRN, the dorsal hippocampus is mostly innervated by the MRN. SSRIs increase extracellular levels of serotonin immediately upon administration [14]. Yet their therapeutic effect is typically delayed for several weeks. This apparent discrepancy may be explained as follows. At least two types of 5-HT autoreceptor are found on the serotonergic neuron. 5-HT_{1A} receptors are present in the somatodendritic area; activation of these receptors decreases neuronal firing, which results in less serotonin being released from the axon terminals. 5-HT_{1B} receptors are located on the terminals of serotonin neurons; when they are activated, serotonin release is directly inhibited. There is growing evidence that postsynaptic 5-HT_{1A} receptors are also involved in the control of serotonin release, through a large feedback loop from terminal to the cell body region [15]. It is very likely that these autorestraining processes counteract the initial effect of SSRIs. Following chronic administration of SSRIs, it has been shown that at least the 5-HT_{1A} receptors (presynaptically as well as postsynaptically) desensitize [16]. Arguably, this adaptive process enhances the effect of the SSRI on serotonergic neurotransmission. This cascade of events may partly explain the delayed onset of action of SSRIs.

Clinical trials: SSRI versus TCA and SSRI versus SSRI

Several meta-analyses of short-term comparative studies have investigated the efficacy of SSRIs compared with TCAs in major depression [17–25]. The majority of these papers did not observe differences in efficacy between the two classes of antidepressant drugs. In one meta-analysis [17], it was found that some TCAs, in particular amitriptyline, may be more effective than SSRIs in depressed patients. A study of combined fluvoxamine data showed that the response rate with this antidepressant was comparable to that seen with tricyclics and tetracyclics [21]. Most short-term, controlled, comparative studies on efficacy did not reveal any differences among the various SSRIs in the treatment of major depression [26–36]. Some studies, however, did find indications for an earlier onset of action of citalopram and paroxetine compared with fluoxetine [28,31,34,36].

Tolerability and long-term efficacy

Several studies have analyzed the adverse-effect profile of SSRIs. In addition to gastro-intestinal effects, headaches and "stimulant adverse effects" like agitation, anxiety, and insomnia were frequently reported [37–42]. Since depression is a chronic recurrent condition, long-term treatment is often required in order to minimize the chance of relapse. Several studies have been performed on relapse during placebo treatment, after initial successful treatment with SSRIs. All studies show that chronic treatment with SSRIs was superior with respect to reappearance of depression and the time to relapse. No evidence was found for differences between SSRIs or between SSRIs and TCAs in terms of relapse features [18,30,42–49]. Although the long-term efficacies of SSRIs and TCAs are similar, the tolerance of SSRIs is clearly superior to TCAs [17,18,22,23,50].

Given the overall limited efficacy in addition to the abundance of side effects a clear need is present for new antidepressants.

Strategies for improvement of antidepressant treatment

Several approaches were used to develop new antidepressants with superior efficacy and tolerability. Some lines have extended current knowledge on monoamines and have focused on more selective uptake inhibitors (escitalopram, reboxetine), dual monoamine uptake inhibition in one compound (duloxetine, venlafaxine, desvenlafaxine, milnacipran, bupropion and hydroxyl bupropion) or triple monoamine uptake inhibition (SEP 225,289 GSK 372,475, DOV 21,947, Tesofensine, JNJ 7925476, PRC 025). Other approaches have used augmentation strategies in an attempt to enhance existing serotonin uptake inhibitor efficacy by adding a functionality that is beneficiary for SSRI biochemistry (SSRI plus moieties). Finally, a plurality of new approaches was explored that are devoid of monoamine uptake inhibition. These approaches use monoaminergic in addition to non-monoaminergic targets.

Ultraselective serotonin uptake inhibitor: escitalopram

Pharmacology of escitalopram

Citalopram and escitalopram represent the latest generation of SSRIs. Citalopram is a racemic mixture of two stereoisomers, R- and S-citalopram. Escitalopram is the S-isomer of citalopram. It was observed in microdialysis and electrophysiological studies in laboratory animals that escitalopram elevates extracellular 5-HT levels in the brain faster and more potently than citalopram. Thus, citalopram is five-times less effective than escitalopram in inhibiting the firing activity of dorsal raphe 5-HT neurons after acute administration [51]. Subacute (3 days) administration of escitalopram leads to the inhibition of firing of norepinephrine (NE) and dopamine (DA) neurons in the rat locus coeruleus (LC) and ventral tegmental area (VTA), respectively [52–54] However, citalopram failed to inhibit NE and DA neurons after subacute administration, even when it was given at 2–4-times higher doses than escitalopram. A microdialysis study by Mork et al. [55] demonstrated that escitalopram produces higher increase in 5-HT levels than the 2-times higher dose of citalopram. It is thus possible that only the S-isomer of citalopram acts as a 5-HT uptake inhibitor, while the R-isomer may partially reverse the 5-HT uptake inhibitory effect of the S-isomer. Indeed, the same study demonstrated that R-citalopram decreases extracellular 5-HT levels. Escitalopram was observed to be very selective in inhibiting the reuptake of serotonin. This compound is currently the most selective SSRI known. Although citalopram was very selective for serotonin reuptake sites, it still had some minor affinities for other receptors. Any affinities for these receptors have been show to be attributable to R-citalopram. Escitalopram is therefore not only the most selective reuptake inhibitor by at least a factor of ten, but also the cleanest. Its pharmacology will therefore be restricted to pure inhibition of the serotonin reuptake site.

Escitalopram in clinical trials

Several clinical trials have been performed to investigate the efficacy of escitalopram in depressed patients. Escitalopram was observed to exert antidepressant activity when compared to placebo in several trials [56–59]. When escitalopram was compared to citalopram, it was shown that escitalopram exerted enhanced effectiveness over citalopram. Escitalopram was observed to induce an earlier onset of action as well as an increased effectiveness in time [60]. Interestingly, a recent study showed that escitalopram was superior to venlafaxine with respect to sustained response and remission [58]. Development of selective, fast-acting and potent 5-HT reuptake inhibitors can be pointed out as one of the directions to improve the efficiency of antidepressant drugs.

Safety and tolerability

The dose of 10 mg/kg of escitalopram was observed to be well tolerated in several clinical trials. Serotonin-related adverse events, such as nausea, sweating, and insomnia, were more frequently present in escitalopram- than in placebo-treated group [56,57]. As the discontinuation rate of escitalopram is not different from placebo, it was investigated whether patients who were intolerable to SSRIs would tolerate escitalopram. Of these patients, 85% were successfully switched to escitalopram, indicative of enhanced tolerability [61].

Selective NE reuptake inhibitors

As with serotonin, a role for NE in depression was suggested by the depressogenic features of reserpine. Abundant evidence is present linking dysfunction of the NE system to depression [62]. In addition, several TCAs are also very potent norepinephrine reuptake inhibitors. The idea that inhibition of norepinephrine uptake, alongside serotonin reuptake inhibition, could be beneficial in treating depression prompted the development of selective norepinephrine reuptake inhibitors, of which reboxetine is currently the only marketed drug.

Reboxetine and the NE system. The noradrenergic system originates mainly in the LC. The α_2-autoreceptors are located on both axon terminals and cell bodies, thus establishing an effective self-regulation system similar to that seen in the serotonergic neuron. Post-mortem studies of the frontal cortex of suicide victims revealed that both the density and affinity of these receptors were increased [50,63]. In addition, α_2-adrenoceptors may become supersensitive during depression [64,65]. Although chronic administration of desimipramine has been shown to effectively reduce the supersensitivity of α_2-adrenoceptors, a recent preclinical study with reboxetine failed to demonstrate changes in receptor function following chronic treatment [64,66]. The β-adrenoceptors are located postsynaptically. Upregulation of these receptors has been observed consistently in patients with depression, whereas downregulation of these receptors is regarded as a marker for antidepressant activity [62]. The relevance of α_2- and β-adrenoceptor downregulation/desensitization for reboxetine's antidepressant effect has yet to be established.

Reboxetine and the 5-HT system. Although the primary target of reboxetine is the NE system, this drug non-directly stimulates 5-HT transmission in the brain. It was reported that chronic administration of reboxetine leads to an increase in the tonic activation of post-synaptic 5-HT$_{1A}$ receptors in the hippocampus [67]. However, the basal firing rate of 5-HT neurons and extracellular 5-HT levels were not affected by reboxetine [66,68].

Reboxetine versus TCAs. Several trials have investigated the efficacy of reboxetine compared with TCAs. In one short-term study, reboxetine was found to be at least as effective as imipramine [69]. Analysis of pooled data from four double-blind outpatient studies also showed no differences between reboxetine and imipramine [70]. Another study comparing imipramine and reboxetine in depressed and dysthymic elderly patients reported better efficacy of reboxetine in dysthymic patients, but not in depressed patients [71,72]. Only one short-term study has compared reboxetine with desimipramine. Equal or superior activity of reboxetine was observed [69].

Reboxetine versus SSRIs. Fluoxetine is the only SSRI that has been compared with reboxetine. Short-term evaluation has shown that the efficacy of reboxetine is similar to fluoxetine [69,73]. Pooling of four double-blind comparison studies, however, revealed increased efficacy of reboxetine compared with fluoxetine in depressed outpatients [70]. Subset analysis on severe depression in several trials showed that reboxetine was superior to fluoxetine [73,74].

Tolerability and long-term efficacy of reboxetine. Reboxetine has been shown to be well tolerated in short-term studies. Adverse events, which have been more frequently observed in reboxetine- versus placebo-treated patients, were dry mouth, constipation, insomnia, increased sweating, tachycardia, vertigo, urinary hesitancy and/or retention, and impotence [75]. Comparison of reboxetine with imipramine and desimipramine revealed a beneficial profile for reboxetine with respect to a number of common side effects like hypotension, dry mouth, and tremor [76,77]. When reboxetine was compared with fluoxetine, patients were observed to be less likely to experience "stimulant adverse effects" as well as gastrointestinal effects [75]. Reboxetine was shown to be effective in the long-term treatment of depression, given its superior efficacy in a one-year placebo-controlled study [69].

Reboxetine in combination with SSRIs. There are several clinical studies demonstrating the efficiency of combined regimen with SSRI and reboxetine in treatment-resistant depression. It can be explained by two possible mechanisms [78,79]. SSRIs stimulate 5-HT transmission by increasing extracellular 5-HT levels; reboxetine may potentiate this effect by sensitization of postsynaptic 5-HT receptors [67]. In addition, the lack of adequate response to SSRIs might be explained, in some patients, by the inhibitory effect of these drugs on NE neuronal activity. Reboxetine possibly reverses the inhibitory effect of SSRIs on NE tone [80].

Dual 5-HT/NE reuptake inhibitors

It was stated above that the combined regimen with 5-HT and NE reuptake inhibitors might be beneficial in depression, and especially in patients resistant to the solo SSRI treatment. Therefore, combining the 5-HT and NE reuptake inhibitory property in the same molecule can provide highly effective antidepressant medication. Indeed, there is evidence that indicates that dual-action uptake inhibitors have enhanced efficacy over single-uptake inhibitors [81]. Currently, several dual-uptake inhibitors are on or close to the market, such as duloxetine, venlafaxine, desvenlafaxine and milnacipran.

Triple 5-HT/NE/DA reuptake inhibitors

Activation of dopaminergic pathways in depressed patients might reverse the symptoms of anhedonia [82]. In line with this observation, nomifensine, which is a potent dopamine uptake inhibitor, was shown to have antidepressant properties [83]. Additionally, bupropion is shown to augment the efficacy of SSRIs in rodents, as well as in humans [84,85]. These observations sparked the development of triple-uptake inhibitors, combining 5-HT, NE, and DA uptake inhibition in a single molecule (SEP 225289, GSK 372475, DOV 21947, NS 2330 (tesofensine), JNJ 7925476, PRC 025 and radafaxine [which is reported to lack 5-HT uptake inhibition]). An obvious liability of dopamine uptake inhibitors is induction of addictive behavior. However, the dynamics of induction of DA inhibition seems to be an important determinant for addiction [86,87]. If this downside of triple-uptake inhibitors can be surpassed, these compounds might induce superior efficacy, but also induce cognitive improvement as well as reduction of sexual side effects [88,89].

DA/NE release stimulator bupropion

Bupropion is an antidepressant and anticraving medication acting as a stimulator of catecholamine (NE and DA) release [90]. This drug showed effectiveness as a monotherapy and as an adjunct to SSRIs.

Targeting specific monoamine receptors with or without serotonin uptake inhibition

The 5-HT$_{1A/1B}$ receptors

An increase in extracellular 5-HT levels by SSRIs leads to the activation of somatodendritic 5-HT$_{1A}$ and nerve-terminal 5-HT$_{1B}$ autoreceptors and to suppression of the firing activity of 5-HT neurons. After several weeks of sustained SSRI administration, the 5-HT neuronal firing activity recovers to the pretreatment levels, due to desensitization of the autoreceptors. It was suggested that the delay between the beginning of the SSRI regimen and onset of the behavioral effects of the treatment might be explained by the 5-HT$_{1A/1B}$ receptor-mediated inhibition of 5-HT neuronal activity. Therefore, blocking 5-HT$_{1A/1B}$ autoreceptors might be beneficial in depression. Agonists of 5-HT$_{1A/1B}$ receptors have also been suggested to be beneficial in depression, since they may facilitate the desensitization of autoreceptors [91,92].

The 5-HT$_{1A/1B}$ receptor-mediated augmentation strategies. Pindolol, a partial agonist of 5-HT$_{1A}$ receptors, has been successfully used as an adjunct to SSRIs in the treatment of depression [93]. It was suggested that the beneficial effect of the thyroid hormone triiodo-thyronine (T3) as an adjunct to TCAs and SSRIs in depression is mediated, at least in part, via 5-HT$_{1B}$ autoreceptors [94].

Therefore, combining 5-HT reuptake inhibitory and 5-HT$_{1A/1B}$ antagonistic properties in one molecule may have therapeutic potential. The combined 5-HT$_{1A}$ reuptake inhibitor and 5HT$_{1A}$ receptor agonist Lu 21004 is currently in phase III of clinical trials. However, the additional 5HT$_3$ antagonistic property of this compound might add to its efficacy [88].

The development of another combined 5-HT$_{1A}$ reuptake inhibitor and 5HT$_{1A}$ receptor agonist, vilazodone, was stopped for development in phase III because of limited clinical efficacy [95].

The 5-HT$_{2A/2C}$ receptors   *Rationale.* It has been observed that blocking of 5-HT$_{2C}$ receptors potentiates the SSRI-induced increase in extracellular 5-HT levels. It suggests the therapeutic potential of 5-HT$_{2C}$ receptor antagonists as adjunct to SSRIs [96]. In addition, the blocking of 5-HT$_{2C}$ receptors reverses the SSRI-induced inhibition of DA neuronal firing activity. Thus, the antagonists of 5-HT$_{2C}$ receptors might be beneficial also due to their ability to prevent the SSRI-induced inhibition of DA transmission [54]. The SSRI-induced inhibition of NE neurons is mediated via 5-HT$_{2A}$ receptors and reversed by 5-HT$_{2A}$ antagonists. Therefore, the beneficial effect of 5-HT$_{2A}$ antagonism on depression may be explained by inhibition or the reversal of tonic or SSRI-induced inhibition of NE neurons [52,53].

The 5-HT$_{2A/2C}$ receptor-mediated augmentation strategies. Agomelatine, an antagonist of 5-HT$_{2C}$ receptors, has been used as solo treatment in depression and as an adjunct to SSRIs [97]. The combined 5-HT$_{2A/2C}$ antagonists nefazodone and mirtazapine showed good efficiency as antidepressant, both in monotherapy or as an adjunct [88]. However, nefazodone has very limited use due to its liver toxicity. All atypical antipsychotic drugs are 5-HT$_{2A}$ and some of them (risperidone) are also 5-HT$_{2C}$ receptor blockers. It may explain their efficiency as mood stabilizers and as adjuncts to SSRIs in depression [52,53].

Therefore, combining 5-HT reuptake inhibition and 5-HT$_{2A/2C}$ antagonism in the same molecule may have great therapeutic potential. One compound, Lu AA 24530, combines these moieties and proved to be efficacious in phase II (www.lundbeck.com).

α$_2$-adrenoceptors   Rationale. Blocking of α$_2$-adrenoceptors stimulates the firing activity of NE neurons and increases extracellular NE levels in the brain. Because of the beneficial role of the stimulation of NE transmission in depression, antagonists of α$_2$-adrenoceptors might be effective antidepressants and/or adjuncts to SSRIs (S39566, R226121) [68,91]. The beneficial effect of some atypical antipsychotic drugs (risperidone) and of mirtazapine may be explained, at least in part, by blocking of α$_2$-adrenoceptors [52,53]. The selective α$_2$-adrenoceptor antagonist idazoxane also showed effectiveness as a mood stabilizer in healthy volunteers [98].

5HT$_{3/5A/7}$ antagonism   Besides the combination of uptake with serotonin receptor type 1 and 2 agonists and antagonists, other serotonin receptors have been investigated as well. Illustrated by the development of Lu21004, 5HT$_3$ antagonism in presence of serotonin uptake inhibition is a logical approach as it reduces SSRI-induced nausea that typically accompanies early treatment with SRIs. The addition of 5-HT$_{5A}$ and 5HT$_7$ antagonism to serotonin uptake inhibition seems promising, yet is currently still in a preclinical stage [99].

Histamine H$_3$ antagonist-SSRI   H$_3$ receptors act as auto- and heteroceptors throughout the brain. Besides the enhanced effects on biochemistry induced by SSRIs, combination of SSRIs with H$_3$ antagonism might also be beneficiary for elevating cognitive dysfunction (JNJ 28583867).

HPA axis-related treatment

Corticotropin-releasing factor (CRF) is secreted from the hypothalamus and has been shown to be involved in the response of organisms to stress [100]. CRF is thought to be hypersecreted from the hypothalamus in depression, which effect is found to occur predominantly via the CRF1 receptor [101,102]. The overproduction of CRF is followed by an overactive hypothalamic–pituitary–adrenal (HPA) axis function, which in turn results in overstimulation of glucocorticoid receptors (GR) [103]. Several approaches are being explored to reduce HPA functionality in depression. One approach is the administration of CRF1 antagonists in order to reduce the central activation of the HPA axis. Pexacerfont, GSK 561679, GSK 586529 and ONO 2333 are examples that are currently in clinical evaluation for efficacy in major depression. Alternatively, the glucocorticoid steroid synthesis inhibitor, metyparone, is also under investigation, as are GR antagonists with SCH 900635 and mefiprestone as examples in phase II.

V1B. In addition to CRF, vasopressin is also involved in regulating HPA axis activity. Vassopressin receptors positively stimulate the adrenocontitropic normone (ACTH) release induced by CRF. This effect is found to be V1B receptor-mediated, which functionally explains the interest in the development of V1B antagonists for depression. SSR 149415, a V1B antagonist is currently in phase II.

Substance P *Rationale.* The neurokinin (NK) substance P (SP) is a peptide found in the central neural system (CNS). There are three types of receptors to SP, SN_{1-3}. All NK receptors are coupled to G-proteins. The main pathways of SP transmission are mediated via SN_1 receptors [104].

There is abundant evidence to support the involvement of SP in depression. First, one of the major functions of SP transmission is pain modulation, as nociception is increased in the majority of depressed patients. Second, there are functional interactions between SP and the monoamine systems. Third, there are SP-related abnormalities that were observed in depressed patients and were reversed by antidepressant treatment, such as increased SP levels in the CSF [105].

Preclinical studies. It was observed in microdialysis studies that the local administration of SP into the DRN increases the 5-HT levels in the DRN and hippocampus and decreases it in the caudate nucleus and PFC. NE levels in the PFC were increased by intra-LC injection of SP. It was thus suggested that SP modulates the activity of 5-HT autoreceptors in the DRN and LC, respectively [105].

Further studies looked into the effect of SSRIs on 5-HT transmission in NK_1-knockout mice or in mice chronically treated with NK_1 blockers. It was found that the effect of paroxetine on extracellular 5-HT levels in the PFC was six-times higher in NK_1 knockout animals and two-and-half-times higher in GR 205171-treated animas than in controls [105].

Electrophysiological studies in laboratory animals suggested that the NK_1 antagonism increases 5-HT transmission via two potential mechanisms: decreasing the sensitivity of $5-HT_{1A}$ autoreceptors in the DRN and stimulating the tonic activation of postsynaptic $5-HT_{1A}$ receptors in the hippocampus [106,107].

There is also evidence on the stimulatory effect of SN_1 antagonism on catecholamine transmission. Microdialysis studies showed the stimulatory effect of GR 205171 on NE levels in the hippocampus [105]. Electrophysiological studies demonstrated that chronic SN_1 antagonists increase the burst activity of NE neurons. A recent study by Haddjeri and Blier [108] demonstrated that 2-day treatment with CP 96345, an antagonist of NK_1 receptors, attenuates the activity of α_2-adrenergic autoreceptors. This study also showed that stimulatory effect of CP 96345 on the firing activity of 5-HT neurons disappeared after lesion of NE system. It can be concluded that NK_1 antagonism stimulates both 5-HT and NE transmission and that its effect on 5-HT system is mediated, at least in part, via NE pathways.

Clinical studies. It was first reported by Kramer et al. [109] that the NK_1 antagonist MK 869 (aprepitant) has an antidepressant effect in humans. This drug is currently in phase III of clinical investigations. Ranga and Krishnan [110] demonstrated that aprepitant has significantly higher clinical efficacy than placebo and comparable efficacy to SSRIs. Combined treatment with SSRIs and NK_1 antagonists may also be a possible clinical strategy; however, it is not yet reported in clinical or preclinical studies. There are also successful attempts to combine 5-HT reuptake inhibition and NK_1 antagonism in one molecule awaiting clinical testing (GSK 424887, S41744).

Acetylcholine Acetylcholine (ACh) is one of the major transmitters in the central, peripheral, and autonomic neuronal system. Brain ACh transmission is mediated via either nicotinic or muscarinic receptors. These are calcium channel and G-protein coupled receptors, respectively. ACh transmission is negatively regulated by ACh esterase (AChE), which metabolizes ACh into choline. Brain ACh plays an important function in learning and memory, synaptic plasticity, neuroprotection, and neuroregeneration [111]. Nicotinic receptors expressed on DA neurons in the VTA increase the responsiveness of DA system to the reward-related stimuli [112].

Since the pathophysiology of depression includes the elements of cognition, learning, neuronal plasticity, and neuroprotection [113], the brain ACh system might be pointed to as one of the potential targets for the treatment of depression.

Clinical studies. The activation of nicotinic receptors may be beneficial in depression, especially in anhedonia, because of the stimulatory effect on DA transmission. However, development of nicotinic receptor-mediated treatment is difficult because of its addictive danger. There are different reports in the literature about the connection between smoking, smoking cessation, and depression [114]. It is interesting that the antidepressant drug bupropion is also an effective anticraving medication in nicotine dependence [115].

The inhibitors of AChE, such as galanthamine, are primarily used in age-related, cognitive and neurodegenerative disorders. Galanthamine is currently in the phase IV of clinical trials in the treatment of Alzheimer and related disorders. A recent study by Elgamal and MacQueen [116,117] showed that galanthamine is also beneficial in depression, as an adjunct to SSRIs. There are also successful attempts to create a medication with combined 5-HT reuptake and AChE inhibitory properties: RS 1259 [118].

Glutamate system *Rationale.* Ionotropic (NMDA) and metabotropic (AMPA) glutamate receptors are shown to be responsible for modulation of mood and related functions that are perturbed in depression [88]. These observations have induced the hypothesis that NMDA and/or AMPA receptors might be targets for the treatment of depression.

NMDA. Blockers of NMDA receptors are under investigation for their antidepressant activity [119]. Although these effects are not uniform, a potent augmentation of antidepressant activity has been described when the NMDA antagonist ketamine is co-administered to depressed patients [120]. CP-101,606 is an example of an antagonist of the NR2B subunit. This specific targeting towards the subunits might circumvent the induction of psychosis and other side effects [88].

AMPA. AMPA receptors are thought to be understimulated compared to NMDA receptors in depression [121]. Positive allosteric modulators of AMPA receptors are under investigation for application in depressive disorders (Org 26576). Likewise, compounds that combine serotonin uptake inhibition with positive allosteric modulation of AMPA receptors are also being studied (LY 392,098 and LY 404,187; [122]).

Gamma-aminobutyric acid (GABA) Several GABA-related approaches are currently being explored. Whereas GABAA stimulation is evaluated, possibly related to its classic facilitation of sleep quality (eszopiclone), other approaches comprise the antagonism of GABAB receptors, which might be precognitive but are also observed to enhance the functionality of SSRIs to elevate 5-HT levels in the PFC [123].

Patients with depression are commonly administered benzodiazepines together with antidepressants. Some studies suggest beneficial effects of benzodiazepines in depressed patients, especially on anxiety and insomnia symptoms [88]. However, a recent study demonstrated that benzodiazepines co-administered with SSRIs diminish the SSRI-induced increase in extracellular 5-HT levels [124]. Thus, the benzodiazepine regimen in depressed patients should be carefully toned.

Table 2.1 Reported clinical development (see www.clinicaltrials.gov or company website).

Cmp	Phase	Company	Activity
Ultraselective uptake inhibitors			
Reboxetine (ss)	II	Pfizer	Norepinephrine uptake inhibitor
Escitalopram	Marketed	Lundbeck	Serotonin uptake inhibitor
Dual action			
Radafaxine	II	GSK	NE/DA uptake inhibitor
DVS-233 (SR) Desvenlafaxine	Marketed	Wyeth	NE/5-HT uptake inhibitor
Bupropion	III	GSK	DA uptake
GSK 372475	II	GSK	Triple-uptake inhibitor (review Millan)
SEP 225, 289	II	Sepracor	Triple-uptake inhibitor
Tesofensine (NS 2330)	II	Neurosearch	Triple-uptake inhibitor
JNJ 7925476	?	J&J	Triple-uptake inhibitor
DOV 21,947	II	DOV Pharmaceutical Inc.	Triple-uptake inhibitor
Armodafinil	II	Cephalon	DA uptake inhibitor
SSRI plus			
Lu AA 21004	III	H. Lundbeck A/S	SSRI/5-HT1A ag/5HT3ant
Vilazodone	II	Merck Darmstadt	SSRI/5-HT1A partial agonist
Lu AA 24530	II	H. Lundbeck A/S	SSRI/5-HT2C antagonist
GW 424887	I	GSK	SSRI/NK1 antagonist
Monoamine receptors			
Agomelatine		Servier	M agonist/5HT2C antagonist
PRX-00023	II	Epix pharma	5-HT1A agonist
GSK 163090	I	GSK	5-HT1A ant
Corticoids/V1B; HPA			
Pexacerfont (BMS 562086)	I/II	BMS	CRF1 antagonist
ONO-2333Ms	II	Ono pharma	CRF1 antagonist
GSK 561679	II	GSK	CRF1 antagonist
586529	I	GSK	CRF1 antagonist
SCH 900636 (org34517)	II	Schering Plough	Glucocorticoid antagonist
Mefiprestone (RU 486)	III	Corcept	Glucocorticoid II antagonist
SSR 149415	II	Sanofi	V1B ant
D2/HT2ant and add ons			
Ropinirole CR		GSK/Stanford	D2/D3 agonist
Antidepressant plus aripiperazole	III	BMS/Otsuka	D2 partial agonist
Quetiapine SR	II	Astra Zeneca	D2/5-HT2 antagonist

Table 2.1 (cont.)

Cmp	Phase	Company	Activity
NK ant			
SR 48968 (saredutant)	III	Sanofi	NK2 antagonist
MK 0869	III	Merck	Aprepitant NK1 ant
AZD 6765	II	AZ	NK1/2 antagonist
GW 597599B	II	GSK	NK1 antagonist
GW 679769	II	GSK	NK1 antagonist
Orvepitant (GW 823296)	I	GSK	NK1 antagonist
GABA agonist			
Eszopiclon	III	Sepracor	GABAA agonist
Cholinergic			
TC-5214 (mecamylamine)	II	Targacept	Nicotine antagonist
RS 1259	II	Sankyo	SRI/esterase inhibitor
Glutamate			
MK-0657	I	Merck	NR2B ant
CP-101,606		Pfizer	NR2B NMDA antagonist
Org 26576	II	Schering Plough	Ampakine
LY 392,098		Eli Lilly	SSRI plus AMPA allo. Fac.
LY 404,187		Eli Lilly	SSRI plus AMPA allo. Fac.
Miscellaneous			
SR 58611 A (amibegron)	III	Sanofi	Beta 3 agonist
Sildenafil	IV	Pfizer	PDE-5 inhibitor
Selegeline transdermal	IV	Somerset	MAOI
SA 4503	II	M's science corp.	Sigma 1 agonist
SSR 411298	II	Sanofi	Fatty acid amide hydrolase inhibitor
Cimicoxib	II	Affectis	COX-2 inhibitor
RG2417	II	Repligen Corp	Uridine
Uridine	II	Repligen Corp	Triacetyluridine
GW 856553X	II	GSK	P38 kinase inhibitor

Miscellaneous   In the quest to generate non-monoaminergic antidepressants, multiple approaches are evaluated. PDE inhibitors might be antidepressants with precognitive properties. Beta 3 agonists, sigma 1 agonists, fatty acid amide hydrolase inhibitors, COX-2 inhibitors, (triacetyl)uridine, and P38 kinase inhibitors all represent diverse approaches that seem promising and await final clinical confirmation in order to evaluate their contribution to antidepressant treatment.

Conclusion

Since the discovery of the relevance of the monoaminergic system in the treatment of depression, most antidepressant treatments have been focused on elevation of central monoamine levels. Now, nearly half a century later, it must be concluded that the abundance of treatments still encompass some sort of stimulatory effect on serotonin, NE and/or DA (selective, dual-and triple-and augmented-uptake inhibitors). Although their clinical efficacy has not increased overwhelmingly, the safety of these compounds certainly has. In addition, as it is realized that depression is a cluster of symptoms rather than a concise disease, approaches target the comorbid features of depression like anxiety, sleep, and cognition. Especially in combination with existing uptake inhibitors, these drugs might turn out to be very potent new generation antidepressants.

It is of further interest that new approaches are increasingly explored (see for example, Table 2.1). Some monoamine ligands that are devoid of uptake inhibition show great promise (agomelatine). Furthermore, non-monoaminergic compounds that are designed to modulate HPA axis, glutamate, GABA, ACl, SP pharmacology are now in phase II and III. Together with approaches such as COX inhibition, PDE inhibitors, beta 3 agonists, sigma 1 agonists, fatty acid amide hydrolase inhibitors, COX-2 inhibitors, (triacetyl)uridine, and P38 kinase inhibitors, a broad array of antidepressant applications are being investigated clinically, providing us with new, non-monoaminergic treatments of depression for the coming century.

References

1. Schildkraut J. J. *Am. J. Psychiatry* 1965; **122**: 509–21.

2. Van Praag H. M., Korf J., Puite J. *Nature* 1970; **225**: 1259–60.

3. Van Praag H. M., Korf J. *Psychopharmacologia* 1971; **19**: 148–52.

4. Sjostrom R. *Eur. J. Clin. Pharmacol.* 1973; **6**: 75–80.

5. Goodwin F. K., Rubovits R., Wehr T. A. *Sci. Proc. Am. Psychiatr. Assoc.* 1977; **130**: 108.

6. Bowers M. B. *J. Nerv. Ment. Dis.* 1974; **158**: 325–30.

7. Faustman W. O., King R. J., Faul K. F., et al. *J. Affect. Disord* 1991; **22**: 235–39.

8. Meltzer H. Y., Lowy M., Robertson A., et al. *Arch. Gen. Psychiatry* 1984; **41**: 391–97.

9. Beskow J., Gottfries C. G., Roos B. E., Winblad D. B. *Acta Psychiatr. Scand.* 1976; **53**: 7–20.

10. Cheetham S. C., Crompton M. R., Czudek C., et al. *Brain Res.* 1989; **502**: 332–40.

11. Woolley D. W., Shaw E. *Science* 1954; **119**: 587–88.

12. Gaddum J. H. *Nature* 1963; **197**: 741–43.

13. Carlsson A, Lindqvist M, Magnusson T. *Nature* 1957; **180**: 1200.

14. Fuller R. W. *Life Sci.* 1994; **55**: 163–67.

15. Bosker F., Vrinten D., Klompmakers A., Westenberg H. *Naunyn Schmiedebergs Arch. Pharmacol.* 1997; **355**: 347–53.

16. Cremers T. I. F. H., Spoelstra E. N., de Boer P., et al. *Eur. J. Pharmacol.* 2000; **397**(2–3): 351–57.

17. Anderson I. M. *Depress. Anxiety* 1998; **7**: 11–17.

18. Anderson I. M., Tomenson B. M. *Br. Med. J.* 1995; **310**: 1433–38.

19. Bech P., Cialdella P. *Int. Clin. Psychopharmacol.* 1992; **6**(Suppl. 5): 45–54.

20. Bech P. In: Dahl S. G., Gram L. F., eds. *Clinical Pharmacology in Psychiatry*. Berlin: Springer, 1989; 81–93.

21. Mendlewicz J. *Drugs* 1992; **43**(Suppl. 2): 32–37.

22. Montgomery S. A., Henry J., McDonald G., et al. *Int. Clin. Psychopharmacol.* 1994; **9**: 47–53.

23. Song F., Freemantle N., Sheldon T. A., et al. *Br. Med. J.* 1993; **306**: 683–87.

24. Steffens D. C., Krishnan K. R., Helms M. J. *Depress. Anxiety* 1997; **6**: 10–18.

25. Tignol J., Stoker M. J., Dunbar G. C. *Int. Clin. Psychopharmacol.* 1992; **7**: 91–94.

26. Aguglia E., Casacchia M., Cassano G. B., et al. *Int. Clin. Psychopharmacol.* 1993; **8**: 197–202.

27. Bennie E. H., Mullin J. M., Martindale J. J. *J. Clin. Psychiatry* 1995; **56**: 229–37.

28. De Wilde J., Spiers R., Mertens C., et al. *Acta Psychiatr. Scand.* 1993; **87**: 141–45.

29. Eskelius L., Von Knorring L., Eberhard G. *Int. Clin. Psychopharmacol.* 1997; **12**: 323–31.

30. Franchini L., Gasperinin M., Perez J., et al. *J. Clin. Psychiatry* 1997; **58**: 104–07.

31. Geretsegger C., Bohmer F., Ludwig M. *Int. Clin. Psychopharmacol.* 1994; **9**: 25–29.

32. Haffmans P. M., Timmerman L., Hoogduin C. A. *Int. Clin. Psychopharmacol.* 1996; **11**: 157–64.

33. Kiev A., Feiger A. J., *Clin. Psychiatry* 1997; **58**: 146–52.

34. Patris M., Bougerol T., Charbonnier J. F., et al. *Int. Clin. Psychopharmacol.* 1996; **11**: 129–36.

35. Rapaport M., Coccaro E., Sheline Y., et al. *J. Clin. Psychopharmacol.* 1996; **16**: 373–78.

36. Tignol J. *J. Clin. Psychopharmacol.* 1993; **13**(Suppl. 2): 18–22.

37. Baldwin D. S., Johnson R. N. *Rev. Contemp. Pharmacother.* 1995; **6**: 315–25.

38. Cooper G. L. *Br. J. Psychiatry* 1988; **15**(Suppl. 3): 77–86.

39. Wagner W., Zaborny B. A., Gray T. E. *Int. Clin. Psychopharmacol.* 1994; **9**: 223–27.

40. Boyer W. F., Blumhardt C. L. *J. Clin. Psychiatry* 1992; **53**(Suppl.): 61–66.

41. Doogan D. P., Caillard V. *Br. J. Psychiatry* 1992; **160**: 217–22.

42. Doogan D. P. *Int. Clin. Psychopharmacol.* 1991; **6**(Suppl. 2): 47–56.

43. Keller M. B., Gelenberg A. J., Hirschfeld R. M., et al. *J. Clin. Psychiatry* 1998; **59**: 598–607.

44. Keller M. B., Kocsis J. H., Thase M. E., et al. *JAMA* 1998; **280**: 1665–72.

45. Montgomery S. A., Dunbar G. C. *Int. Clin. Psychopharmacol.* 1993; **8**: 189–95.

46. Montgomery S. A., Henry J., McDonald G., et al. *Int. Clin. Psychopharmacol.* 1994; **9**: 47–53.

47. Montgomery S. A., Kasper S. *Int. Clin. Psychopharmacol.* 1995; **9**(Suppl. 4): 33–40.

48. Robert P., Montgomery S. A. *Int. Clin. Psychopharmacol.* 1995; **10**(Suppl. 1): 29–35.

49. Rush A. J., Koran L. M., Keller M. B., et al. *J. Clin. Psychiatry* 1998; **59**: 589–97.

50. Meana J. J., Barturen F., Garcia-Sevilla J. A. *Biol. Psychiatry* 1992; **1**: 471–90.

51. El Mansari M., Sánchez C., Chouvet G., Renaud B., Haddjeri N. *Neuropsychopharmacology* 2005; **30**(7): 1269–77.

52. Dremencov E., El Mansari M., Blier P. *J. Psychiatry Neurosci.* 2009; **34**(3): 223–29.

53. Dremencov E., El Mansari M., Blier P. *Psychopharmacology (Berl).* 2007; **194**(1) : 63–72. Epub 2007 May 27.

54. Dremencov E., El Mansari M., Blier P. *Biol. Psychiatry* 2007; **61**(5): 671–78. Epub 2006 Aug 24.

55. Mork A., Kreilgaard M., Sanchez C., Brennum L. T., Wiborg O. *CINP* 2002. P.1.E.054. Montreal.

56. Wade A., Lemming O., Hedegaard K. B., Poster presented at Scandinavian College of Neuropsychopharmacology (SCNP) 1st Annual Meeting April 18–21, 2001, Juan les Pins, France.

57. Lepola U., Loft H., Reines E. H. Poster presented at Scandinavian College of Neuropsychopharmacology (SCNP) 1st Annual Meeting, April 18–21, 2001, Juan les Pins, France.

58. Montgomery S. A. 2002 Press release (7–10–2002, no. 81).

59. Burke W. J. Poster presented at Scandinavian College of Neuropsychopharmacology (SCNP) 1st Annual Meeting, April 18–21, 2001, Juan les Pins, France.

60. Gorman J. Poster presented at the 11th Annual Meeting of the Association of European Psychiatrists, May 4–8, 2002, Stockholm.

61. Rosenthal M., Zornberg G., Li D. *CINP* 2002. P.3.E.038. Montreal.

62. Leonard B. E. J. *Psychopharmacology* 1997; **11**(Suppl. 4): S39–47.

63. Callado L. F., Meana J. J., Grijalba B., et al. *J. Neurochem.* 1998; **70**: 1114–23.

64. Charney D. S., Heninger G. R., Sternberg D. E., et al. *Arch. Gen. Psychiatry* 1981; **38**: 1334–40.

65. Spyraki C., Fibiger H. C. *Life Sci.* 1980; **27**: 1863–67.

66. Sacchetti G., Bernini M., Bianchetti A., et al. *Br. J. Pharmacol.* 1999; **128**(6): 1332–38.

67. Szabo S. T., Blier P. *Neuropsychopharmacology* 2001; **25**(6): 845–57.

68. Szabo S. T., Blier P. *Eur. J. Neurosci.* 2001; **13**(11): 2077–87.

69. Montgomery S. A. *J. Psychopharmacol.* 1997; **11**(Suppl. 4): S9–15.

70. Massana J., Moller H. *Proc. Ann. Meeting. Am. Psychiatr Assoc.*, Toronto, Canada 1998.

71. Dubini A., Bosc M., Polin V. J. *Psychopharmacology* 1997; **11**(Suppl. 4): S17–23.

72. Katona C., Bercoff E., Chiu E., et al. *J. Affect. Disord.* 1999; **55**: 203–13.

73. Massana J. *J. Clin. Psychiatry* 1998; **59**(Suppl. 14): 8–10.

74. Montgomery S. A. *Int. J. Psychiatry Clin. Pract.* 1999; **3**(Suppl. 1): S13–17.

75. Mucci M. *J. Psychopharmacol.* 1997; **11**: S33–37.

76. Ban T. A., Gaszner P., Aguglia E., et al. *Hum. Psychopharmacol.* 1998; **13**: 529–39.

77. Berzewski H., van Moffaert M., Gagiano C. A. *Eur. Neuropsychopharmacol.* 1997; **7**(Suppl. 1): S37–47.

78. López-Muñoz F., Alamo C., Rubio G., García-García P., Pardo A. *Pharmacopsychiatry* 2007; **40**(1): 14–19.

79. Fava M. *J. Clin. Psychiatry* 2000; **61**(Suppl 1): 26–32.

80. Tremblay P., Blier P. *Curr. Drug Targets* 2006; **7**(2): 149–58.

81. Thase M. E., Nierenberg A. A., Keller M. B., Panagides J. *J. Clin. Psychiatry* 2001; **62**(10): 782–88.

82. Nestler E. J., Carlzon W. A. *Biol. Psychiatry* 2006; **59**: 1151–59.

83. Corrigan M. H., Denahan A. Q., Wright C. E., Ragual R. J., Evans D. L. *Depression Anxiety* 2000; **11**: 58–65.

84. Prica C., Hascoet M., Bourin M. *Behav Brain Res.* 2008; **194**: 92–99.

85. Axford L., Booth J. R., Hotten T. M., et al. *Bioorg. Med. Chem. Lett.* 2003; **13**: 3277–80.

86. Samaha A. N., Robinson T. E. *Trends Pharmacol. Sci.* 2005; **26**: 82–87.

87. Volkow N. D., Wang G. J., Fowler J. S., et al. *Biol. Psychiatry* 2005; **57**: 640–46.

88. Millan M. J. *J. Pharmacol. Exp. Ther.* 2006; **110**: 135–370.

89. El-Ghundi M., O'Dowd B. F., George S. R. *Rev. Neurosci.* 2007; **18**: 37–66.

90. Dong J., Blier P. *Psychopharmacology (Berl.)* 2001; **155**: 52–57.

91. Mongeau R., Blier P., de Montigny C. *Brain Res. Brain Res. Rev.* 1997; **23**: 145–95.

92. Blier P., Piñeyro G., el Mansari M., Bergeron R., de Montigny C. *Ann. NY Acad. Sci.* 1998; **861**: 204–16.

93. Portella M. J., de Diego-Adeliño J., Puigdemont D., et al. *Eur. Neuropsychopharmacol.* 2009; **19**: 516–19.

94. Lifschytz T., Segman R., Shalom G., et al. *Curr. Drug Targets* 2006; **7**(2): 203–10.

95. De Paulis T. *IDrugs* 2007; **10**: 193–201.

96. Cremers T. I., Giorgetti M., Bosker F. J., et al. *Neuropsychopharmacology* 2004: **29**(10): 1782–89.

97. Goodwin G. M., Emsley R., Rembry S., Rouillon F., for the Agomelatine Study Group. *J. Clin. Psychiatry.* Epub 2009 Aug 11.

98. Coupland N. J., Bailey J. E., Wilson S. J., Potter W. Z., Nutt D. J. *Clin. Pharmacol. Ther.* 1994; **56**: 420–29.

99. Thomas D. R., Soffin E. M., Roberts C., et al. *Neuropharmacology* 2006; **51**: 566–77.

100. Arborelius L., Owens M. J., Plotsky P. M., Nemeroff C. B. *J. Endocrinol.* 1999; **160**: 1–12.

101. Lovenberg T. W., Liaw C. W., Grigoriadis D. E., et al. *PNAS* 1995; **92**: 836–40.

102. Chalmers D. T., Lovenberg T. W., De Souza E. B. *J. Neurosci.* 1995; **15**: 6340–50.

103. Gold P. W., Chrousos G. P. *Mol. Psychiatry* 2002; **7**: 254–75.

104. Van der Hart M. *Substance P and the Neurokenin 1 Receptor.* Groningen, Netherlands, Ipskamo Drukkers BV, 2009.

105. Guiard B. P., Lanfumey L., Gardier A. M. *Curr. Drug Targets* 2006; **7**: 187–201.

106. Gobbi G., Blier P. *Peptides* 2005; **26**: 1383–93.

107. Blier P., Gobbi G., Haddjeri N., et al. *Psychiatry Neurosci.* 2004; **29**: 208–18.

108. Haddjeri N., Blier P. *Eur. J. Pharmacol.* 2008; **600**(1–3): 64–70.

109. Kramer M. S., Cutler N., Feighner J., et al. *Science* 1998; **281**: 1640–45.

110. Ranga K., Krishnan R. *J. Clin. Psychiatry* 2002; **63**(Suppl. 11): 25–29.

111. McKay B. E., Placzek A. N., Dani J. A. *Biochem. Pharmacol.* 2007; **74**: 1120–33.

112. Mansvelder H. D., Mertz M., Role L. W. *Semin. Cell Dev. Biol.* 2009; **20**: 432–40.

113. Dremencov E., Gur E., Lerer B., Newman M. E. *Prog. Neuropsychopharmacol. Biol. Psychiatry*, 2003; **27**(5): 729–39.

114. Ischaki E., Gratziou C. *Ther. Adv. Respir. Dis.* 2009; **3**: 31–38.

115. Lising-Enriquez K., George T. P. *J. Psychiatry Neurosci.* 2009; **34**: E1–2.

116. Elgamal S., MacQueen G. *J. Clin. Psychopharmacol.* 2008; **28**: 357–59.

117. Elgamal S. A., Marriott M., Macqueen G. M. *J. Clin. Neurophysiol.* 2009; **26**: 192–97.

118. Abe Y., Aoyagi A., Hara T., et al. *J. Pharmacol. Sci.* 2003; **93**: 95–105.

119. Zarate C. A., Singh J. B., Quiroz J. A., et al. *Am. J. Psychiatry* 2006; **163**: 153–55.

120. Zarate C. A., Zing J. B., Carlson P. J., et al. *Arch. Gen. Psychiatry* 2006; **63**: 856–64.

121. Maeng S., Zarate C. A., Du J., et al. *Biol. Psychiatry* 2008; **63**: 349–52.

122. Black M. D. *Psychopharmacology* 2005; **179**: 154–63.

123. Rea K., Dremencov E., Cremers T.I.F.M., et al. Augmentation of citalopram response by antagonists of γ-amino-butyric type-B (GABA) receptors. *Psychopharmacology* 2010; forthcoming.

124. Cremers T.I.F.M., Dremencov E., Bosker F. J., et al. Benzodiazepines diminish paroxetine-induced elevation of serotorin levels in guinea pig hippocampus *Int. J. Neuropsychopharmacol* 2010; forthcoming.

Developing novel animal models of depression

Lotte de Groote, Malgorzata Filip, and Andrew C. McCreary

Abstract

Although the mechanism of action of current antidepressant drugs is well known, 30% of patients remain refractory to treatment. There are examples of recent failures of antidepressant clinical development programs that reinitiate the discussion on the reliability, or predictability of animal models of major depressive disorder. The comorbid expression of depression is well known in many neurological and psychiatric diseases, including drug abuse. Symptoms such as anhedonia, hypo- or hyperlocomotor activity, sleep disturbances, and weight loss can be measured in animals, but the overreliance on such readouts may lead to misinterpretations of their relevance to the clinical situation. Existing models are mainly based, or could be considered to have an overreliance, on the putative involvement of monoaminergic systems. Data recorded from these existing models do result in clinical candidate nomination, but when such compounds reach the clinic, data often do not fully meet expectations. From a preclinical point of view, the integration of the range of established and novel technologies, such as monitoring dynamic changes in extracellular neurotransmitters, behavioral readouts, electrophysiological recordings, and brain scanning (e.g. using functional magnetic resonance imaging and spectroscopy, PET, SPECT imaging) is critically needed in the development of new animal models, as is the translation of such approaches to the clinic and vice versa. This integration is needed across the gamut of indication areas of key interest.

Introduction

Depression is one of the most prevalent psychiatric disorders and has unfavorable prognosis and suicide risk [1–3]. Depression is more common in women than men, with a lifetime prevalence of about 10% and 20%, respectively [4,5]. Despite the currently available antidepressants, about one-third of depressive patients do not respond to pharmacotherapy, and full remission is only achieved in a third of patients. Clearly, improved efficacy of pharmacotherapeutic intervention is needed in order to alleviate the personal and socio-economic burdens of this debilitating disease.

The therapeutic action of antidepressants drugs was first recognized in the 1950s with the use of tricyclic antidepressants (e.g. imipramine) which block the reuptake of serotonin (5-hydroxytryptamine; 5-HT) and norepinephrine, but also have off-target effects at muscarinic and histamine receptors. Monoamine oxidase (MAO) inhibitors are effective antidepressants, and although compounds acting on MAO-B are relatively safe, those having efficacy at MAO-A often interact with dietary tyramine, eliciting a pressor response. In the 1980s selective 5-HT reuptake inhibitors (SSRI; e.g. fluvoxamine, fluoxetine, citalopram)

Next Generation Antidepressants: Moving Beyond Monoamines to Discover Novel Treatment Strategies for Mood Disorders, ed. Chad. E. Beyer and Stephen M. Stahl. Published by Cambridge University Press.
© Cambridge University Press 2010.

were introduced followed by a serotonin/norepinephrine reuptake inhibitor (SNRI; e.g. reboxetine) or combined SSR/NRI approaches (e.g. venlafaxine), and while better tolerated than the "classical" medications they do have similar clinical response rates. Antidepressants with novel mechanisms of action include tianeptine, a 5-HT reuptake enhancer [6,7], and agomelatine, a 5-HT2C receptor antagonist and melatonin-1/2 receptor agonist [8,9], and have shown promise in the clinical efficacy setting. For example, tianeptine demonstrated superiority to reference comparators (to tricyclic antidepressants and SSRI) in clinical studies [10,11].

Despite the high prevalence, the etiology of depression remains unclear, making the accurate delineation of animal models difficult. Moreover, the clinical manifestation of depression is heterogeneous and often complicated by comorbid expression of anxiety traits [12,13]. Besides the risk of suicide, patients suffering from depression also present somatic diseases including coronary heart disease, type 2 diabetes, obesity [14,15], and chronic pain [16]. If patients do respond to current antidepressant medication, the latency to clinical efficacy is often 4–6 weeks. This delayed effect is clearly of clinical importance, as ineffectiveness and side effects in this period often have negative impact and discontinuation of the therapy is common [17], or in some cases may lead to suicide [18,19]. While the mechanism of action of antidepressant drugs has been studied extensively over the past 30 years, it remains unclear what causes the delay in onset of action, as current drugs targeting monoaminergic reuptake and degradation are able to increase levels of monoamines immediately after acute administration [20]. Recently, 5-HT reuptake inhibition combined with blockade of 5-HT1A somatodendritic autoreceptors was thought to mimic a gradual desensitization process resulting in a faster onset of therapeutic action. Pindolol, a non-selective 5-HT1A/beta-adrenoceptor antagonist, accelerated the clinical effect of an SSRI [20,21], a hypothesis which has collected much debate since that time. However, more recent double-blind placebo-controlled studies have not verified this hypothesis [22,23].

Additional hypotheses suggest that changes in postsynaptic 5-HT1A, 5-HT2A, and 5-HT2C receptor changes are crucial (for detailed reviews see [24–26]). Promising novel antidepressant drug targets include the neuropeptidergic systems. However, after negative results in multicenter double-blind placebo-controlled studies with the neurokinin-1 antagonist aprepitant [27], this concept has been largely abandoned for the pharmacotherapy of depression. While a large body of evidence still exists for a role of corticotropin-releasing factor (CRF) receptors in stress-related depression [28–30], so far clinical trials with antagonists for these receptors have resulted in limited evidence for clinical efficacy [31]. Multitarget drugs, targeting several neurotransmitter or peptidergic systems, have been suggested as potentially better antidepressant drugs [32–34].

The lack of novel but more importantly improved pharmacotherapies for depression and other psychiatric disorders is far from trivial [35–38]. Existing animal models of depression have primarily been designed to show efficacy of "monoaminergic type" of antidepressants and therefore may not predict clinical efficacy of drugs with novel mechanisms of action [34,39]. Importantly, non-pharmacological treatments of depressive symptoms are effective ranging from psychotherapy and exercise in milder forms of depression to electroconvulsive therapy, vagus nerve stimulation, and deep brain stimulation for severely depressed patients [40–43] and even placebo treatment [44,45]. Given the clinical heterogeneity of depression, a multidisciplinary approach to explore the neurobiological bases for the many subtypes of depression is therefore essential [46]. On face values the development of novel models of depression might appear trivial, but developing an animal model for a disease with unknown etiology is an extremely complex task. New genetic technologies facilitate comparisons between species and systems, and recent advances in in-vivo brain monitoring techniques such as magnetic resonance imaging (MRI) and SPECT make it possible to visualize brain abnormalities in humans and small rodents. These exciting developments have translational potential to contribute to our understanding of depression and modeling relevant symptoms in animals with validity for antidepressant treatment. In this chapter we discuss behavioral models and symptoms of depression and their brain correlates as potential translational approaches to be used in developing novel animal models and potential pitfalls in the modeling of depression in the non-clinical environment.

Clinical symptoms of depression

Depression is often chronic, episodic, and with high risk of recurrence. Major depressive disorder is characterized by an abnormal depressed mood (dysphoria) and loss of pleasure from natural rewards (anhedonia). This blunted affect is present for most of the day, with a duration of at least two weeks. In addition, there are a number of other symptoms causing marked functional impairment, such as psychomotor retardation and agitation sleep disturbance (insomnia or hypersomnia), lack of energy, poor concentration, a lack or increase in appetite, recurrent morbid thoughts about death, and suicidal ideation [47]. However, signs of these symptoms and their severity may be very different between patients. Depression is a clinically heterogeneous disorder, which underscores the disease complexity. Whereas the etiology of depression remains unclear, depressive mood is certainly not limited to clinical (major) depressive disorder, but is also part of bipolar, other mood disorders, psychiatric (e.g. schizophrenia) and neurological disorders (e.g. Parkinson's disease). Moreover, following withdrawal from abused drugs, a syndrome consisting of depressive symptoms is one of the most commonly described. Depression is described after withdrawal from the psychostimulants amphetamine and cocaine [48], nicotine [49], opiate [50], alcohol [51,52], and phencyclidine in humans. Antidepressants can attenuate symptoms of withdrawal of drugs of abuse [53,54], suggesting, at least in part, that the symptoms could resemble signs of endogenous depression.

In addition to the core symptoms of the disease, stress is an important factor in depression [55,56]. Hyperactivity of the hypothalamic–pituitary–adrenal (HPA) axis is one of the most consistent biological findings in major depression, but the mechanisms underlying this abnormality remain unclear [57]. Importantly, dysfunction of the HPA axis system are involved in the development and course of depression [58].

Depressive symptoms modeled in animals

A detailed knowledge of the clinical etiology of depression, and related disorders, is necessary in order to try and model the disease condition. The etiology of depression remains poorly understood. The monoamine deficiency hypothesis of depression was introduced over 30 years ago, and since then research has been stirred by several other hypotheses of depression involving corticosteroid receptors [55,59], neuroimmunology [60,61], neurogenesis [62,63], neuroplasticity [64–67], and epigenetics [68].

A limitation in a preclinical model is that not all depression criteria can be modeled in laboratory animals. Assessing depressed mood or thoughts about death or guilt are obviously limited to humans. Also, the wide spectrum of disruptions characteristic of depression are impossible to model in a single laboratory animal model of the disorder. Therefore, a gamut of models likely needs to be employed in order to build an accurate picture of efficacy. According to the primary definition by McKinney and Bunney in 1969, an animal model of depression should attempt to mimic the human disorder in its manifestation or symptomatology (face validity), a change in the animal's behavior should be monitored objectively, the behavioral changes should be reversed by the same treatment modalities that are effective in humans (predictive validity), and the change should be reproducible between investigators [69]. Geyer and Markou postulated that the animal model should have only strong predictive validity while the behavioral readout should be reliable and robust within and between laboratories [70]. Further, these authors suggested that construct or discriminant validity are not essential for basic neurobiological research and drug discovery [70,71]. Thus, modeling a core symptom or endophenotype rather than syndromal modeling of the disease state is needed, and to increase predictability of variables these need to be translated from the patient to the animal, but importantly then also back to the patient. Anhedonia as a core symptom can be modeled in animals, although reduced hedonia is not a symptom exclusively seen in depression but is also a key symptom in schizophrenia [47]. In animals anhedonia is inherently difficult to measure, but is commonly measured as sucrose intake or as rates of intracranial self-stimulation [72]. Disturbed sleep, appetite, bodyweight, hypoactivity (psychomotor symptoms) can be easily assessed in animals. However, abnormalities of these physiological measures by themselves do not predict a depressive-like phenotype per se.

Current animal models of depression

The focus in drug discovery is typically on animal models that are predictive of efficacy and safety in humans. Animal models of depression have been extensively reviewed (e.g. see refs. [71–75]). Many approaches have been attempted, for example, neurochemical or lesion-based models, ethological models based on social or environmental stress, stress coping response, or genetic manipulation, and while Table 3.1 is not exhaustive, it illustrates the variety of existing animal models of depression and we draw on these for illustration purposes.

The forced swim test (FST), as originally described by Porsolt and colleagues, is probably the most widely used behavioral procedure for assessing antidepressant activity in rodents [77,78]. It is a 1–2 day procedure in which animals swim under conditions from which escape is not possible. In the FST, a rat or a mouse is placed in a cylinder filled with water of varying water temperature. Initially the animal tries to escape until it gives up and displays immobility, a floating position. When using rats, the FST is conducted over 2 days with the test compound applied on the second day, whereas, for unknown reasons, in mice a single FST exposure is enough to reveal antidepressant-like effects. Whereas tricyclic antidepressants and SNRI drugs were effective, the original model in the rat developed by Porsolt did not reveal antidepressant activity of SSRIs [79]. A modification of the FST was needed to demonstrate that the increased depth of water in the swimming tank resulted in less immobility displayed by animals and revealed differential effects on struggling and swimming behavior by noradrenergic and serotonergic antidepressant drugs, respectively [80,81]. This nicely illustrates how a pitfall (false negative) in an original test was overcome by making some experimental adjustments and sharpening behavioral observations, but at the same time also shows how the behavioral response of animals is influenced by experimental procedures. However, in the FST, using a procedure whereby animals swim in cold water results in hypothermia of the animal, but using warmer water (30–35 °C) increases floating behavior and does not allow discrimination of antidepressant drug effects in a number of laboratories. Hypothermia may interfere with drug effects; therefore, a test was developed in mice based on an inescapable situation, but without

Table 3.1 Animal models of depression.

Preclinical paradigm	References
Antidepressant-like	
forced swim test (FST)	[77,78]
modified forced swim test	[81]
tail suspension test (TST)	[73]
differential reinforcement of low-rate 72-s schedule	[99]
Stress	
learned helplessness	[100]
prenatal stress	[102–104]
chronic mild stress	[93,104]
chronic social stress (tree shrews)	[105]
social defeat (or resident-intruder)	[106,108]
maternal deprivation (social isolation)	[109]
Drug	
drug-withdrawal-induced anhedonia	[98,110]
neonatal clomipramine, neonatal SSRI	[111,112]
Lesion	
olfactory bulbectomy	[113,114]
Genetic	
modified mice	[73]
5-HT transporter knockout rat	[115]
Flinders-sensitive line rats	[116,117]
congenital learned helpless rats	[107,118]
high and low anxiety rats and mice	[119,120]
"Rouen mouse" (TST)	[76,121]

use of water. In the tail suspension test (TST), mice are suspended by their tails (using adhesive tape) and positioned nose-down from a rod, creating a situation from which they cannot escape, and similar to the FST immobility time is scored. The response to stress or situation from which an animal cannot escape triggers mechanisms that may, or at least have been hypothesized to, be related to symptoms of depression. Behavioral immobility in the FST and TST allows for adaptive retraction from the inescapable stress of forced swimming or tail suspension and comprises a coping strategy [82] in which immobility behaviors represent the psychological concept of "entrapment" (arrested flight) described in clinical depression [83]. Primarily, FST and TST are used to detect the effects of antidepressant drugs (a shorter immobility time or a longer latency to immobility than control injection means antidepressant-like action). In addition, recent evidence shows that increased immobility or a shortened latency to immobility in the above tests are associated with depressive-like behavior or with the negative symptoms of schizophrenia, i.e. avolition [84–88]. Increased immobility in the FST is found in animals during early life or prenatal stressors, genetic alteration in noradrenergic or opioid receptors, the postpartum state, deprivation of tryptophan in diet, withdrawal from abused drugs, and is seen in other models of depression, such as the Flinders rat model, neonatal clomipramine administration, social isolation, olfactory bulbectomy, learned helplessness, chronic mild stress (see for references Table 3.1, [99–121]). Strain differences in the response to antidepressant drugs have been described for rat (Long–Evans, Sprague–Dawley, Wistar, Wistar–Kyoto; [89,90] and mouse (e.g. BALB/cJ, C57/B6, DBA/2J, DBA/2Ha, FVB/NJ, NMRI, NIH-Swiss; [73,91,92]. Whereas assessing immobility time (FST and TST) may seem simple behavioral scores, testing should be performed with caution, as the outcome of these tests can be very much influenced by procedural differences, including differences in animal strains used, notably in mice, but differences in rats have also been demonstrated [74]. In the unpredictable chronic mild stress model, animals are exposed to mild forms of stress such as reversal of the light/dark cycle, tilted cage, wet bedding, and social isolation during a period of several weeks up to two months (type and number of stressors and duration depends on the laboratory). Models using mild forms of stress are preferred, as chronic stressors involving pain such as electric foot shock or tail pinch are considered unethical. Over the years the chronic mild stress procedure has had difficulties in reproducibility, and therefore its reliability is sometimes questioned [71,74,93].

The clinical picture of withdrawal caused by known drugs of abuse was readily translated to laboratory animals [94,95]. Moreover, as in humans, antidepressants can attenuate symptoms of drugs of abuse withdrawal in rats [54,96]. Abuse drug (e.g. amphetamine) withdrawal displays high levels of predictive and construct validity [97]; however, it should be stressed that it is difficult to model all symptoms of such withdrawal using one animal model [98]. In addition, the designs of drug treatment (dose, route, number of injections, duration between injections, time of behavioral readouts relative to drug exposure) are important factors determining the subsequent different behavioral effects in rodents. Several drugs of abuse (psychostimulants, opioids, ethanol, nicotine, phencyclidine) produce a depressive-like phenotype on withdrawal, but notably the anhedonic state of rats produced by these drugs is proportional to the amount of drug consumed as well as its pattern of administration. On the other hand, it seems that the motivational aspects of drug intake are not important for withdrawal effects, as both voluntary (i.e. active drug administration in self-administration models) and passive (by an experimenter) drug administration produced anhedonic states in rodents. The time of treatment is another important factor; however, withdrawal from drugs of abuse offers only a narrow window to study depression (effects seen up to 5–14 withdrawal days). Taken together, behavioral results suggest that the applicability of withdrawal to drugs of abuse as a model of human endogenous depression has limitations, given the transient nature of the depressive symptoms and complications of type of drug administration schedule used.

Novel animal models of depression?

In the past decade, overwhelming numbers of genetic mouse models with depressive-like phenotype have been described (see ref. [73] for a review of depressive-like behaviors in about 40 strains of modified mice). Single gene mutations are certainly useful to study the mechanism of novel (drug) targets in the absence of selective pharmacological tools. Nevertheless, complex disorders like depression and other psychiatric illness are unlikely due to a single gene deficit. As pointed out by many others, it should be emphasized not to anthropomorphize animal behavior [122,123] and that an animal with a molecular defect shows behavioral characteristics that may be associated with depression in humans.

Response to chronic antidepressant treatment mimics the clinical situation; however, this latency to effect is not often covered in the animal models. On the other hand, if chronic antidepressants are effective, this is not necessarily a model of depression. For example, in the novelty-induced hypophagia model selective effects of chronic fluoxetine are observed [124]. In contrast to acute novelty suppressed feeding tests in food-deprived animals, in this hypophagia model animals are first trained to novel food, then tested in their home cage and the following day anxiety behavior is measured in a novel environment. Chronic SSRI treatment was effective in the novelty-induced hypophagia model, and this finding is in line with the effectiveness of chronic SSRIs in human anxiety disorders [125,126]. On the other hand, the novelty-induced hypophagia model may also be thought of as a "hybrid model," as in addition to being a test of anxiety, this model is sensitive to chronic (but not acute) antidepressants [75]. In attempts to create new experimental paradigms, variations on an existing test can, however, be made. For example, refinement of the original Porsolt paradigm with extended behavioral analyses or even repeated forced swimming in a larger pool (i.e. a classical Morris water maze test to study learning and memory without a hidden platform) was found to induce immobility behavior in rats, which was reversed by chronic antidepressant treatment [127,128]. Unlike the FST, this open-space swim test takes place over 3 test days, and animals are thought to develop escape strategies that could be indicative of cognitive capacity [129], which are also impacted in depression. The Morris water maze is a classical test of spatial reference memory thought to be a hippocampal-dependent cognitive task [130]. Interestingly, recent modifications of this test showed that working memory and reverse learning could be assessed, and these cognitive behaviors were affected by stress hormone-induced prefrontal cortex (PFC) abnormalities [131]. Reverse learning in the water maze, as a measure of behavioral flexibility, was impaired in rats subjected to unpredictable chronic mild stress and could be reversed by antidepressants [132].

Stress response

Like humans, individual animals also differ in their response to stressors [133,134]. These individual differences to stressors and stress susceptibility can be used to select animals with a depressive-like behavior. For example, in a model of stress-induced anhedonia, chronic stress (alternate exposure to restraint stress for rat, and tail suspension) induced anhedonia in a subset of mice, while the remaining animals did not show a hedonic-like deficit or other depressive-like behaviors. Strikingly, chronic treatment with an SSRI was selectively effective in animals with a hedonic deficit [135]. Individual stress susceptibility can be induced by subjecting adolescent mice to a highly unstable social environment, a chronic stressor with regular changes in the group composition. Susceptible mice showed an altered stress response later on in life, and some aspects (body fat composition) of these changes were prevented by antidepressant treatment during the chronic stress exposure [136,137].

Individual differences in a population can be taken for selective breeding of animals with a high or low response to a certain stimulus resembling a depressive-like response. For example, selective breeding with high and low responders to anxiety-related behavior (elevated plus maze and a variety of other tests) resulted in an enhanced depression-like FST behavior in the high anxiety rats, an effect prevented by chronic treatment with the SSRI paroxetine [138,139]. Other models include mice selected for immobility response by the TST [121], congenital learned helplessness [107], and restraint stress [110]. However, the weakness of such approaches is the requirement for generations of selective breeding (e.g. 29 generations in the aforementioned line of congenital learned helplessness rats) before a picture emerges whether one extreme of the selection indeed models a "depressed" animal. Taken together, animal models based on individual susceptibility to stressors may be crucial, not only to study subtypes of depression, but also those of comorbidities such as anxiety and substance abuse. Stress is also a well-known risk factor in substance abuse [140,141]. Animal models based on social stress may be very useful for disorders of mood and drug addiction, especially since various types of social stress have their own behavioral and physiological profile relevant to subtypes of clinical symptoms [142,143].

Gender differences

Despite the fact that the prevalence of clinical depression is twice as high in females as males, there is an enormous gap of information from preclinical models in females. Gender differences in clinical depression and response to psychotropic medication are well recognized [5,144]. There is also evidence of differences between male and female rats in their response to controllability and antidepressant treatment [145]. In the FST, naïve female animals showed more immobility than males, and the response to imipramine affected the behavioral response depending on the phase of the female estrous cycle [146]. Despite a differential profile in the FST between genders, with decreased immobility latency and increased climbing duration in females, the tricyclic antidepressant clomipramine was overall as effective in females as in males [147]. In many models of depression it is unknown whether females respond differently to antidepressant treatment when compared to males.

Gender differences in animal models of depression and anxiety have, however, been described [148]. Sucrose intake, as a measure of anhedonia, in the olfactory bulbectomy model was lower in female rats compared to males [149]. In the learned helplessness model of depression, animals display helplessness in response to uncontrollable stress; however, females failed to develop this behavior [150]. Female animals were found to be more vulnerable to chronic mild stress than males (as reflected in reduced sucrose intake, higher stress hormone levels, and decreased serotonergic activity in the hippocampus), but in contrast to males these stressed females showed less immobility behavior in the FST [151]. Housing conditions in social animals like rats or mice are important for behavioral effects to stressors. For example, when housed socially, chronic stressed female rats showed enhanced stress coping behaviors [152]. Social isolation is stressful to rats and caused a specific hippocampal plasticity response in female Flinders-sensitive rats, a rat strain displaying depressive-like behavior, but not in female control rats [153]. Females have higher circulating levels of corticosterone and greater HPA axis responsiveness to stress [154]. Surprisingly, in a recent microdialysis study, free corticosterone levels in the brain showed no gender difference under baseline conditions, and only a subtle gender difference in response to acute swim stress [155]. Research on the mechanisms underlying the differential vulnerability of the stress coping response and to antidepressant treatments in females versus males is vital to understanding gender differences in depression.

Brain changes in depression

Looking "into the brain" of depressed patients by means of in-vivo neuroimaging have revealed structural, functional, and chemical abnormalities [156,157]. Visualizing these brain abnormalities with non-invasive techniques ideally comprise follow-up studies on treatment effects, comparison to non-depressed controls, and can be applied easily to any age group.

Understanding these brain abnormalities in depression is important to increase our knowledge of the etiology and furthermore could serve, in the future, as potential diagnostic criteria, or at least biomarkers, of depressive symptoms. Methods used to monitor in-vivo changes in the brain are PET and SPECT (receptor–ligand interactions, glucose metabolism, drug distribution), functional magnetic resonance imaging (fMRI; blood flow and oxygenation) and magnetic resonance spectroscopy (MRS) can be used to quantify levels of certain neurochemicals and metabolites. Structural imaging and post-mortem studies in brains of depressed patients have shown reductions in gray matter volume of hippocampus and PFC [156]. Both the hippocampus and PFC are key brain areas thought to mediate cognitive aspects of depression. Moreover, the hippocampus is an important brain structure involved in behavioral and neuroendocrine responses to stress [158,159]. The hippocampus is also an important target of 5-HT and norepinephrine neurotransmission affected by antidepressants [160], and of molecular changes in response to antidepressants and stress [161,162]. Other brain areas likely to be involved include the nucleus accumbens, amygdala, and certain hypothalamic nuclei, and are critical in responses to rewarding and aversive stimuli and regulating motivation, eating, sleeping, energy level, circadian rhythm, which are all abnormal in depressed patients [163].

Abnormalities in brains of patients with depression as demonstrated with in-vivo brain imaging techniques include altered metabolism in specific brain areas, abnormal balance within brain circuits, and changes in amino acid neurotransmitters and other brain chemicals. Many functional imaging studies in depressed patients using fluoro-2-deoxyglucose-PET or fMRI have found altered metabolic rates of glucose in the PFC, cingulate cortex, and amygdala. Mayberg proposed an abnormal balance in limbic stress/emotion regions based on neuroimaging observations in depressive patients [164]. Dorsal cortical brain regions control executive function, attention, cognitive processes, whereas motivated behaviors mediated by the ventral limbic system are more involved in expression of emotions, aversion, stress, and negative affect. During depression or "induced sadness," a shift in neuronal activity (as measured by blood flow or glucose metabolism) was observed with decreases in the cortical brain regions and increases in limbic stress/emotion regions [165,166]. Moreover, this shift in brain activity could be reversed by antidepressant treatments [165]. Depressed patients showed increased activity particularly in the subgenual anterior cingulate cortex, a node of interaction between the stress and positive cortical networks. Deep brain stimulation of the subgenual anterior cingulate cortex relieves depressive symptoms in otherwise treatment-resistant patients [40].

MRS can detect a variety of brain chemicals such as the putative neuronal marker N-acetylaspartate, levels of choline-containing compounds in astroglial cells, and the energy metabolites creatine and phosphocreatine in all cells. The so-called glutamix signal consists of a combined spectrum of glutamate, glutamine, and GABA. Glutamate–glutamine cycling flux between neurons and glia is vital to glutamatergic neurotransmission. Unfortunately the low intrinsic sensitivity limits glutamate and GABA signals to some brain regions like the frontal and occipital cortices; however, the monitoring of these amino acids may become available in the human hippocampus with higher field strengths and further technical improvements in MRS techniques. Post-mortem studies and notably in-vivo MRS imaging have provided evidence for involvement of glutamate and other amino acid neurotransmitters in the pathophysiology and treatment of mood disorders. Glial cell abnormalities associated with mood disorders may at least partly account for the impairment in glutamate action since glial cells play a primary role in synaptic glutamate removal [167]. Lower glutamine/glutamate levels have consistently been found in the cortex of depressive patients [168], and after prefrontal electro-convulsive therapy (ECT) these levels, and also those of N-acetylasparate, choline, and creatine were increased in patients [169,170]. Further support for a role of glutamate comes from a recent study demonstrating a fast-acting antidepressant effect of ketamine, an antagonist at the glutamatergic N-methyl-D-aspartic acid (NMDA) receptor in treatment-resistant major depression. Patients reported significant improvement on the day and lasting up to one week after ketamine was administered [171]. Although the mechanism is not fully understood, it is an exciting finding that a drug can have a fast antidepressant effect. MRS studies have revealed abnormal GABA concentrations in several neuropsychiatric disorders including epilepsy, anxiety disorders, major depression, and drug addiction [172]. Low GABA in occipital and anterior cingulate cortices of unmedicated, acutely depressed patients has been reported [173], and these reduced GABA levels were increased after antidepressants and ECT [174,175]. Studies in unmedicated but recovered patients suggest that lower prefrontal GABA levels may indicate vulnerability for recurrent depression [176]. GABA receptors are, however, difficult to target directly, due to the side effects of sedation and hypothermia, although allosteric modulation of the GABA-B receptor could have therapeutic potential [177].

Dopamine and the reward system are heavily associated with drug abuse, but may also be linked to depression [178]. Anhedonia and psychomotor symptoms appear to be mediated by dopaminergic mesolimbic and mesostriatal projections, the key brain systems affected by psychostimulant drugs. Metabolic changes are observed in the brains of cocaine and meth-amphetamine abusers as shown by decreased glucose metabolism (2FDG-PET) in the anterior cingulate and orbitofrontal cortices [179]. PET studies in abusers of these psycho-stimulant drugs consistently showed reduced monoaminergic transporter density and reduced dopamine D2 receptors in striatal regions, reduced N-acetylasparate and total creatine in the basal ganglia, as well as altered brain glucose metabolism that correlated with severity of psychiatric symptoms in the limbic and orbitofrontal regions [178].

Importantly, like in human studies, in-vivo brain imaging should provide examples of follow-up studies in animal models for the monitoring of treatment effect within subjects. Moreover, in addition to brain scanning, the non-invasive methods allow also the assessment of a behavioral readout within the same subject, thereby strengthening correlations of neurochemical changes with behavioral symptoms.

In-vivo brain monitoring in animal models of depression

Non-invasive imaging techniques in small animals have great translational potential. Whereas the strength in human MRI studies is within functional imaging studies, a caveat is that animals need to be lightly anesthetized to avoid unwanted movements during the scan. While spatial and temporal resolutions are improving magnetic resonance technology (with recent reports showing submillimeter resolution in fMRI signals at present), both temporal and spatial resolution for PET are suboptimal at present [180]. In small laboratory animals fMRI can be used to define circuits of drug action. MRI has been applied in rodents to investigate drugs of abuse and some psychotropic drugs, including NMDA antagonists [181–183]. Preliminary effects of antidepressant drugs on blood oxygenation signal are now reported [184]. Beyond these "drug signature" types of studies in normal animals, applying pharmaco-MRI could be promising for defining affected brain circuitry in animal models of depression and therefore correlating this to clinical findings. In addition to MRI,

PET can be applied to study experimental manipulation in the whole brain, whereas other techniques allow in-vivo monitoring from distinct brain regions of interest. So far, limited studies have used MRS to study in-vivo changes in neurotransmitters and their metabolites in animal models of depression. Closest to human MRS findings are probably studies on the psychosocial stress model in tree shrews. In this animal model, social stress (exposure of a subordinate to dominant animals) reduced the in-vivo brain concentrations of N-acetyl-aspartate, total creatine, and choline-containing compounds, an effect that could be reversed by chronic treatment with different antidepressant drugs [185,186]. Choline and creatine signals may reflect changes in energy metabolism and glial function. In learned helplessness rats, elevated creatine levels were found after ECT [187]. This finding was in line with a study by the same authors in depressed patients, where they showed increases in creatine after ECT [187]. Moreover, in learned helplessness rats, elevated glutamate/GABA signals in the hippocampus and PFC were found after ECT [188]. A drawback of MRS is that it is as yet an expensive technique, limiting its application in preclinical animal research; moreover, it is limited to certain brain chemicals and is not applicable for all types of neurotransmitters. Brain imaging in animal models generates high expectations, but ultimately the application of new novel techniques needs to prove their added value.

A powerful technique in animals is in-vivo microdialysis, an invasive technique that allows sampling in distinct brain regions from awake and freely moving animals. Liquid chromatography combined with mass spectroscopy or electrochemical detection, and radio-immunoassays are generally used to quantify extracellular neurotransmitters and neuro-peptides with high selectivity and sensitivity in dialysate. Microdialysis studies have greatly contributed to our understanding of the mechanisms of action of psychoactive drugs including antidepressants and their influence on monoaminergic, cholinergic, and amino acid systems [189,190]. Complementary to microdialysis, enzyme-based biosensors are thought to have high potential for the measurement of transmitters such as glutamate with high time resolution [191]. Biosensor techniques can also be applied for monitoring brain metabolism (brain tissue oxygen and glucose); however, studies relevant to depression are not available as yet. Whereas in-vivo microdialysis is used extensively to determine the mechanism of antidepressant drug action, limited studies have been performed in animal models of depression. Examples of in-vivo neurochemical changes in some models of depression are reported. In olfactory bulbectomized rats, less 5-HT was available for release in the hippocampus and amygdala, but 5-HT synthesis capacity was unaffected [192]. In the ventral striatum of bulbectomized rats, significantly higher basal dopamine and lower norepinephrine levels were found. These dopaminergic abnormalities could correlate to the hyperactive behavior of olfactory bulbectomized animals in response to an open field [192]. In the chronic mild stress model, lower hippocampal GABA levels were observed in the stress exposed animals [193]. The latter finding in a rat model fits with clinical data of altered GABA-ergic function in depressed patients [173]. In the PFC and nucleus accum-bens, chronic mild stress affected dopamine responsiveness to motivational and aversive stimuli (food and tail pinch stress, respectively), suggesting motivational and possibly learning deficits in these stressed rats [194].

Recent PET studies in rats showed reduced dopamine D2/3 receptor binding in the dorsal striatum of amphetamine exposed animals, a finding consistent with clinical studies in drug abusers [179]. The mesolimbic system, the dopaminergic projections from the ventral tegmental area to the nucleus accumbens, is well known for its role in reward but may extend to motivational processes and depression-like symptoms [178]. Changes in several monoaminergic and GABA-ergic neurotransmitter systems in depression were recognized to show similarities to those of drug withdrawal of psychostimulants [96]. Microdialysis studies in the nucleus accumbens in rats after drug withdrawal demonstrated decreased glutamate, and increased GABA and dopamine levels [96]. Future in-vivo neurochemical studies may further support clinical findings focused on the prefrontal and orbitofrontal brain regions, and are of particular interest to unravel the prefrontal glutamate–nucleus accumbens pathway in motivation and drug of abuse-related changes [195].

In rats subjected to the FST, brain region-specific responses of norepinephrine and 5-HT levels to the second swim exposure were found, as were differential effects to antidepressant drugs [196,197]. While the coping behaviors in the forced swim may be considered psychological stress, forced swimming is also a strong physiological stressor (hypothermia), as reflected in the substantial increase in levels of free corticosterone in the hippocampus [145]. An important but confounding factor is the water temperature, and it should be taken into account that during forced swimming at 25 °C the core body temperature of the rat decreases by about 8 °C [198]. Water temperature determines the neurochemical response of GABA, 5-HT and its metabolite 5-HIAA in the hippocampus, and also the behavioral responses to forced swim stress [198,199]. Hippocampal levels of GABA were decreased in response to acute swim stress, whereas when the water temperature was close to the rat's body temperature a small increase in GABA was found [199]. Taken together, cautious interpretation of forced swim data-based procedures regarding the underlying neurochemical "antidepressant" response is needed.

Concluding remarks

In the research process animal models are needed to predict the efficacy and safety of novel drugs in humans. As listed in Table 3.2, shortcomings in the development of novel and in existing animal models for depression include overlooking individual variability, differences between animal strains, and gender. Depression is a complex heterogeneous disease and requires experimental models to differentiate subtypes and comorbidities. This is a major pitfall in the discovery of novel antidepressant treatment, since many of the animal models have an overreliance on the monoaminergic hypotheses of depression. Such an overreliance on these hypotheses may lead to misinterpretation/misprediction of the potential of the true efficacy of the clinical testing scenario. Refinement of existing animal models is therefore pivotal to our understanding of the disease and improved pharmacotherapy. In this respect,

Table 3.2 Pitfalls in animal models of depression.

Procedure or model to detect antidepressant-like effect
Modeling disease or symptoms
Chronic versus acute drug administration
Individual variability
Species differences
Sex differences
Strain differences
Coupling of behavioral and brain correlates

the animal models and the use of a wider spectrum of methods and measures including biomarkers and non-invasive in-vivo brain monitoring methods that provide an insight into aberrant neurochemical parameters coupled with behavioral phenotypic identification could improve the translational aspects of depression modeling.

References

1. Wittchen, H. U., Knauper, B., and Kessler, R. C. 1994, *Br. J. Psychiatry Suppl*, 16.

2. Ebmeier, K. P., Donaghey, C., and Steele, J. D. 2006, *Lancet*, **367**, 153.

3. Bernal, M., Haro, J. M., Bernert, S., et al. 2007, *J. Affect. Disord.*, **101**, 27.

4. Paykel, E. S. 1991, *Br. J. Psychiatry Suppl*, 22.

5. Piccinelli, M. and Wilkinson, G. 2000, *Br. J. Psychiatry*, **177**, 486.

6. Wilde, M. I. and Benfield, P. 1995, *Drugs*, **49**, 411.

7. Kasper, S. and McEwen, B. S. 2008, *CNS Drugs*, **22**, 15.

8. den Boer, J. A., Bosker, F. J., and Meesters, Y. 2006, *Int. Clin. Psychopharmacol.*, **21** Suppl 1, S21.

9. Olie, J. P. and Kasper, S. 2007, *Int. J. Neuropsychopharmacol.*, **10**, 661.

10. Invernizzi, G., Aguglia, E., Bertolino, A., et al. 1994, *Neuropsychobiology*, **30**, 85.

11. Waintraub, L., Septien, L., and Azoulay, P. 2002, *CNS Drugs*, **16**, 65.

12. Kaufman, J. and Charney, D. 2000, *Depress. Anxiety*, **12** Suppl 1, 69.

13. Kessler, R. C., Berglund, P., Demler, O., et al. 2003, *JAMA*, **289**, 3095.

14. Evans, D. L., Charney, D. S., Lewis, L., et al. 2005, *Biol. Psychiatry*, **58**, 175.

15. Farmer, A., Korszun, A., Owen, M. J., et al. 2008, *Br. J. Psychiatry*, **192**, 351.

16. Millan, M. J. 1999, *Prog. Neurobiol.*, **57**, 1.

17. van Geffen, E. C., van der Wal, S. W., van, Hulten R., de Groot, M. C., Egberts, A. C., and Heerdink, E. R. 2007, *Eur. J. Clin. Pharmacol.*, **63**, 1193.

18. Hirschfeld, R. M., Keller, M. B., Panico, S., et al. 1997, *JAMA*, **277**, 333.

19. Trivedi, M. H., Hollander, E., Nutt, D., and Blier, P. 2008, *J. Clin. Psychiatry*, **69**, 246.

20. Artigas, F., Romero, L., de, Montigny C., and Blier, P. 1996, *Trends Neurosci.*, **19**, 378.

21. Blier, P. 2001, *J. Clin. Psychiatry*, **62** Suppl 15, 12.

22. Perry, E. B., Berman, R. M., Sanacora, G., Anand, A., Lynch-Colonese, K., and Charney, D. S. 2004, *J. Clin. Psychiatry*, **65**, 238.

23. Geretsegger, C., Bitterlich, W., Stelzig, R., Stuppaeck, C., Bondy, B., and Aichhorn, W. 2008, *Eur. Neuropsychopharmacol.*, **18**, 141.

24. Hjorth, S., Bengtsson, H. J., Kullberg, A., Carlzon, D., Peilot, H., and Auerbach, S. B. 2000, *J. Psychopharmacol.*, **14**, 177.

25. Millan, M. J. 2005, *Therapie*, **60**, 441.

26. Cremers, T. I., Rea, K., Bosker, F. J., et al. 2007, *Neuropsychopharmacology*, **32**, 1550.

27. Keller, M., Montgomery, S., Ball, W., et al. 2006, *Biol. Psychiatry*, **59**, 216.

28. Nemeroff, C. B. 1992, *Neuropsychopharmacology*, **6**, 69.

29. Arborelius, L., Owens, M. J., Plotsky, P. M., and Nemeroff, C. B. 1999, *J. Endocrinol.*, **160**, 1.

30. Reul, J. M. and Holsboer, F. 2002, *Curr. Opin. Pharmacol.*, **2**, 23.

31. Holsboer, F. and Ising, M. 2008, *Eur. J. Pharmacol.*, **583**, 350.

32. Millan, M. J. 2006, *Pharmacol. Ther.*, **110**, 135.

33. Berton, O. and Nestler, E. J. 2006, *Nat. Rev. Neurosci.*, **7**, 137.

34. Conn, P. J. and Roth, B. L. 2008, *Neuropsychopharmacology*, **33**, 2048.

35. Spedding, M., Jay, T., Costa e Silva, J. and Perret, L. 2005, *Nat. Rev. Drug Discov.*, **4**, 467.

36. Agid, Y., Buzsaki, G., Diamond, D. M., et al. 2007, *Nat. Rev. Drug Discov.*, **6**, 189.

37. Markou, A., Chiamulera, C., Geyer, M. A., Tricklebank, M., and Steckler, T. 2008, *Neuropsychopharmacology*, **34**, 74.

38. Sams-Dodd, F. 2006, *Drug Discov. Today*, **11**, 355.

39. Henn, F. A., Edwards, E., Anderson, D., and Vollmayr, B. 2002, *World Psychiatry*, **1**, 115.

40. Mayberg, H. S., Lozano, A. M., Voon, V., et al. 2005, *Neuron*, **45**, 651.

41. Nemeroff, C. B., Mayberg, H. S., Krahl, S. E., et al. 2006, *Neuropsychopharmacology*, **31**, 1345.

42. Nemeroff, C. B. 2007, *J. Psychiatr. Res.*, **41**, 189.

43. Johansen-Berg, H., Gutman, D. A., Behrens, T. E., et al. 2008, *Cereb. Cortex*, **18**, 1374.

44. Walsh, B. T., Seidman, S. N., Sysko, R., and Gould, M. 2002, *JAMA*, **287**, 1840.

45. Zimmerman, M., Posternak, M. A., and Ruggero, C. J. 2007, *J. Clin. Psychopharmacol.*, **27**, 177.

46. Krishnan, V. and Nestler, E. J. 2008, *Nature*, **455**, 894.

47. American Psychiatric Association 1994, *Diagnostic and Statistical Manual of Mental Disorders* (fourth edition). Washington, DC, American Psychiatric Press.

48. Pathiraja, A., Marazziti, D., Cassano, G. B., Diamond, B. I., and Borison, R. L. 1995, *Prog. Neuropsychopharmacol. Biol. Psychiatry*, **19**, 1021.

49. Hughes, J. R., Gust, S. W., Skoog, K., Keenan, R. M., and Fenwick, J. W. 1991, *Arch. Gen. Psychiatry*, **48**, 52.

50. Haertzen, C. A. and Hooks, N. T., Jr. 1969, *J. Nerv. Ment. Dis.*, **148**, 606.

51. Grant, B. F. and Harford, T. C. 1995, *Drug Alcohol Depend.*, **39**, 197.

52. Gilman, S. E. and Abraham, H. D. 2001, *Drug Alcohol Depend.*, **63**, 277.

53. Gawin, F. H., Kleber, H. D., Byck, R., et al. 1989, *Arch. Gen. Psychiatry*, **46**, 117.

54. Markou, A., Hauger, R. L., and Koob, G. F. 1992, *Psychopharmacology (Berl)*, **109**, 305.

55. Holsboer, F. 2000, *Neuropsychopharmacology*, **23**, 477.

56. McEwen, B. S. 2003, *Biol. Psychiatry*, **54**, 200.

57. Pariante, C. M. and Lightman, S. L. 2008, *Trends Neurosci.*, **31**, 464.

58. Muller, M. B. and Holsboer, F. 2006, *Biol. Psychiatry*, **59**, 1104.

59. McEwen, B. S. 2000, *Brain Res.*, **886**, 172.

60. Dunn, A. J., Swiergiel, A. H., and de Beaurepaire, R. 2005, *Neurosci. Biobehav. Rev.*, **29**, 891.

61. Anisman, H., Merali, Z., and Hayley, S. 2008, *Prog. Neurobiol.*, **85**, 1.

62. Nestler, E. J., Gould, E., Manji, H., et al. 2002, *Biol. Psychiatry*, **52**, 503.

63. Duman, R. S. and Monteggia, L. M. 2006, *Biol. Psychiatry*, **59**, 1116.

64. Duman, R. S., Heninger, G. R., and Nestler, E. J. 1997, *Arch. Gen. Psychiatry*, **54**, 597.

65. Fuchs, E., Czeh, B., Kole, M. H., Michaelis, T., and Lucassen, P. J. 2004, *Eur. Neuropsychopharmacol.*, **14** Suppl 5, S481.

66. Matthews, K., Christmas, D., Swan, J., and Sorrell, E. 2005, *Neurosci. Biobehav. Rev.*, **29**, 503.

67. Castren, E. 2005, *Nat. Rev. Neurosci.*, **6**, 241.

68. Tsankova, N. M., Berton, O., Renthal, W., Kumar, A., Neve, R. L., and Nestler, E. J. 2006, *Nat. Neurosci.*, **9**, 519.

69. McKinney, W. T., Jr. and Bunney, W. E., Jr. 1969, *Arch. Gen. Psychiatry*, **21**, 240.

70. Geyer, M. A. and Markou, A. 2002, *Neuropsychopharmacology: The Fifth Generation of Progresss*, Nashville, TN, American College of Neuropsychopharmacology, 445.

71. Cryan, J. F., Markou, A., and Lucki, I. 2002, *Trends Pharmacol. Sci.*, **23**, 238.

72. Carlezon, W. A., Jr. and Chartoff, E. H. 2007, *Nat. Protoc.*, **2**, 2987.

73. Cryan, J. F. and Mombereau, C. 2004, *Mol. Psychiatry*, **9**, 326.

74. McArthur, R. and Borsini, F. 2006, *Pharmacol. Biochem. Behav.*, **84**, 436.

75. Kalueff, A. V., Wheaton, M., and Murphy, D. L. 2007, *Behav. Brain Res.*, **179**, 1.

76. El Yacoubi, M. and Vaugeois, J. M. 2007, *Curr. Opin. Pharmacol.*, **7**, 3.

77. Porsolt, R. D. 1979, *Biomedicine*, **30**, 139.

78. Porsolt, R. D., Le Pichon, M., and Jalfre, M. 1977, *Nature*, **266**, 730.

79. Borsini, F. 1995, *Neurosci. Biobehav. Rev.*, **19**, 377.

80. Detke, M. J., Rickels, M., and Lucki, I. 1995, *Psychopharmacology (Berl)*, **121**, 66.

81. Cryan, J. F., Page, M. E., and Lucki, I. 2005, *Psychopharmacology (Berl)*, **182**, 335.

82. Thierry, B., Steru, L., Chermat, R., and Simon, P. 1984, *Behav. Neural Biol.*, **41**, 180.

83. Gilbert, P. and Allan, S. 1998, *Psychol. Med.*, **28**, 585.

84. Velazquez-Moctezuma, J. and Diaz Ruiz, O. 1992, *Pharmacol. Biochem. Behav.*, **42**, 737.

85. Woods-Kettelberger, A., Kongsamut, S., Smith, C. P., Winslow, J. T., and Corbett, R. 1997, *Expert. Opin. Investig. Drugs*, **6**, 1369.

86. Hansen, H. H., Sanchez, C., and Meier, E. 1997, *J. Pharmacol. Exp. Ther.*, **283**, 1333.

87. Tizabi, Y., Rezvanil, A. H., Russell, L. T., Tyler, K. Y., and Overstreet, D. H. 2000, *Pharmacol. Biochem. Behav.*, **66**, 73.

88. Noda, Y., Kamei, H., Mamiya, T., Furukawa, H., and Nabeshima, T. 2000, *Neuropsychopharmacology*, **23**, 375.

89. Vetulani, J., Nalepa, I., and Popik, P. 1991, *Pol. J. Pharmacol. Pharm.*, **43**, 187.

90. Lopez-Rubalcava, C. and Lucki, I. 2000, *Neuropsychopharmacology*, **22**, 191.

91. Petit-Demouliere, B., Chenu, F., and Bourin, M. 2005, *Psychopharmacology (Berl)*, **177**, 245.

92. Calcagno, E., Canetta, A., Guzzetti, S., Cervo, L., and Invernizzi, R. W. 2007, *J. Neurochem.*, **103**, 1111.

93. Willner, P. 1997, *Psychopharmacology (Berl)*, **134**, 319.

94. Leith, N. J. and Barrett, R. J. 1980, *Psychopharmacology (Berl)*, **72**, 9.

95. Kokkinidis, L. and Zacharko, R. M. 1980, *Psychopharmacology (Berl)*, **68**, 73.

96. Markou, A., Kosten, T. R., and Koob, G. F. 1998, *Neuropsychopharmacology*, **18**, 135.

97. Barr, A. M. and Markou, A. 2005, *Neurosci. Biobehav. Rev.*, **29**, 675.

98. Murphy, C. A., Fend, M., Russig, H., and Feldon, J. 2001, *Behav. Neurosci.*, **115**, 1247.

99. O'Donnell, J. M., Marek, G. J., and Seiden, L. S. 2005, *Neurosci. Biobehav. Rev.*, **29**, 785.

100. Maier, S. F. 1984, *Prog. Neuropsychopharmacol. Biol. Psychiatry*, **8**, 435.

101. Newport, D. J., Stowe, Z. N., and Nemeroff, C. B. 2002, *Am. J. Psychiatry*, **159**, 1265.

102. Morley-Fletcher, S., Darnaudery, M., Mocaer, E., et al. 2004, *Neuropharmacology*, **47**, 841.

103. Weinstock, M. 2008, *Neurosci. Biobehav. Rev.*, **32**, 1073.

104. Papp, M., Moryl, E., and Willner, P. 1996, *Eur. J. Pharmacol.*, **296**, 129.

105. van Kampen, M., Kramer, M., Hiemke, C., Flugge, G., and Fuchs, E. 2002, *Stress*, **5**, 37.

106. Kudryavtseva, N. N. 2000, *Neurosci. Behav. Physiol.*, **30**, 293.

107. Vollmayr, B. and Henn, F. A. 2001, *Brain Res. Brain Res. Protoc.*, **8**, 1.

108. Buwalda, B., Kole, M. H., Veenema, A. H., et al. 2005, *Neurosci. Biobehav. Rev.*, **29**, 83.

109. Lehmann, J., Pryce, C. R., Jongen-Relo, A. L., Stohr, T., Pothuizen, H. H., and Feldon, J. 2002, *Neurobiol. Aging*, **23**, 457.

110. Barr, A. M., Markou, A., and Phillips, A. G. 2002, *Trends Pharmacol. Sci.*, **23**, 475.

111. Vogel, G., Neill, D., Hagler, M., and Kors, D. 1990, *Neurosci. Biobehav. Rev.*, **14**, 85.

112. Maciag, D., Williams, L., Coppinger, D., and Paul, I. A. 2006, *Eur. J. Pharmacol.*, **532**, 265.

113. Song, C. and Leonard, B. E. 2005, *Neurosci. Biobehav. Rev.*, **29**, 627.

114. Roche, M., Shanahan, E., Harkin, A., and Kelly, J. P. 2008, *Pharmacol. Rep.*, **60**, 404.

115. Olivier, J. D., Van Der Hart, M. G., Van Swelm, R. P., et al. 2008, *Neuroscience*, **152**, 573.

116. Overstreet, D. H. 1993, *Neurosci. Biobehav. Rev.*, **17**, 51.

117. Overstreet, D. H., Friedman, E., Mathe, A. A., and Yadid, G. 2005, *Neurosci. Biobehav. Rev.*, **29**, 739.

118. Chourbaji, S., Zacher, C., Sanchis-Segura, C., Dormann, C., Vollmayr, B., and Gass, P. 2005, *Brain Res. Brain Res. Protoc.*, **16**, 70.

119. Landgraf, R., Wigger, A., Holsboer, F., and Neumann, I. D. 1999, *J. Neuroendocrinol.*, **11**, 405.

120. Touma, C., Bunck, M., Glasl, L., et al. 2008, *Psychoneuroendocrinology*, **33**, 839.

121. Vaugeois, J. M., Odievre, C., Loisel, L., and Costentin, J. 1996, *Eur. J. Pharmacol.*, **316**, R1.

122. Crawley, J. N. and Paylor, R. 1997, *Horm. Behav.*, **31**, 197.

123. Holmes, P. V. 2003, *Crit. Rev. Neurobiol.*, **15**, 143.

124. Dulawa, S. C. and Hen, R. 2005, *Neurosci. Biobehav. Rev.*, **29**, 771.

125. Zohar, J. and Westenberg, H. G. 2000, *Acta Psychiatr. Scand. Suppl.*, **403**, 39.

126. Baldwin, D. S., Anderson, I. M., Nutt, D. J., et al. 2005, *J. Psychopharmacol.*, **19**, 567.

127. Sun, M. K. and Alkon, D. L. 2003, *J. Neurosci. Methods*, **126**, 35.

128. Schulz, D., Buddenberg, T., and Huston, J. P. 2007, *Neurobiol. Learn. Mem.*, **87**, 624.

129. Sun, M. K. and Alkon, D. L. 2006, *J. Pharmacol. Exp. Ther.*, **316**, 926.

130. Kesner, R. P. 2000, *Hippocampus*, **10**, 483.

131. Cerqueira, J. J., Pego, J. M., Taipa, R., Bessa, J. M., Almeida, O. F., and Sousa, N. 2005, *J. Neurosci.*, **25**, 7792.

132. Bessa, J. M., Mesquita, A. R., Oliveira, M., et al. 2009, *Front. Behav. Neurosci.*, **3**, 1.

133. Henn, F. A. and Vollmayr, B. 2005, *Neurosci. Biobehav. Rev.*, **29**, 799.

134. Crowley, J. J. and Lucki, I. 2005, *Curr. Pharm. Des.*, **11**, 157.

135. Strekalova, T., Gorenkova, N., Schunk, E., Dolgov, O., and Bartsch, D. 2006, *Behav. Pharmacol.*, **17**, 271.

136. Sterlemann, V., Ganea, K., Liebl, C., et al. 2008, *Horm. Behav.*, **53**, 386.

137. Schmidt, M. V., Czisch, M., Sterlemann, V., Reinel, C., Samann, P., and Muller, M. B. 2008, *Stress*, **12**, 89.

138. Landgraf, R. and Wigger, A. 2002, *Behav. Genet.*, **32**, 301.

139. Muigg, P., Hoelzl, U., Palfrader, K., et al. 2007, *Biol. Psychiatry*, **61**, 782.

140. Kreek, M. J. and Koob, G. F. 1998, *Drug Alcohol Depend.*, **51**, 23.

141. Weiss, F. 2005, *Curr. Opin. Pharmacol.*, **5**, 9.

142. Koolhaas, J. M., Korte, S. M., de Boer, S. F., et al. 1999, *Neurosci. Biobehav. Rev.*, **23**, 925.

143. Miczek, K. A., Yap, J. J., and Covington, H. E., III. 2008, *Pharmacol. Ther.*, **120**, 102.

145. Leuner, B., Mendolia-Loffredo, S., and Shors, T. J. 2004, *Biol. Psychiatry*, **56**, 964.

144. Gorman, J. M. 2006, *Gend. Med.*, **3**, 93.

146. Barros, H. M. and Ferigolo, M. 1998, *Neurosci. Biobehav. Rev.*, **23**, 279.

147. Kokras, N., Antoniou, K., Dalla, C., et al. 2009, *J. Psychopharmacol.*, **23**, 945.

148. Palanza, P. 2001, *Neurosci. Biobehav. Rev.*, **25**, 219.

149. Stock, H. S., Ford, K., and Wilson, M. A. 2000, *Pharmacol. Biochem. Behav.*, **67**, 183.

150. Dalla, C., Edgecomb, C., Whetstone, A. S., and Shors, T. J. 2008, *Neuropsychopharmacology*, **33**, 1559.

151. Dalla, C., Antoniou, K., Drossopoulou, G., et al. 2005, *Neuroscience*, **135**, 703.

152. Westenbroek, C., Ter Horst, G. J., Roos, M. H., Kuipers, S. D., Trentani, A., and den Boer, J. A. 2003, *Prog. Neuropsychopharmacol. Biol. Psychiatry*, **27**, 21.

153. Bjornebekk, A., Mathe, A. A., Gruber, S. H., and Brene, S. 2007, *Hippocampus*, **17**, 1193.

154. Kudielka, B. M. and Kirschbaum, C. 2005, *Biol. Psychol.*, **69**, 113.

155. Droste, S. K., de, Groote L., Atkinson, H. C., Lightman, S. L., Reul, J. M., and Linthorst, A. C. 2008, *Endocrinology*, **149**, 3244.

156. Drevets, W. C. 2001, *Curr. Opin. Neurobiol.*, **11**, 240.

157. Mayberg, H. S. 2003, *Br. Med. Bull.*, **65**, 193.

158. Meijer, O. C. and De Kloet, E. R. 1998, *Crit. Rev. Neurobiol.*, **12**, 1.

159. Carrasco, G. A. and Van de Kar, L. D. 2003, *Eur. J. Pharmacol.*, **463**, 235.

160. Mongeau, R., Blier, P., and de Montigny, C. 1997, *Brain Res. Brain Res. Rev.*, **23**, 145.

161. Duman, R. S., Malberg, J., and Nakagawa, S. 2001, *J. Pharmacol. Exp. Ther.*, **299**, 401.

162. Fuchs, E., Czeh, B., and Flugge, G. 2004, *Behav. Pharmacol.*, **15**, 315.

163. Nestler, E. J., Barrot, M., DiLeone, R. J., Eisch, A. J., Gold, S. J., and Monteggia, L. M. 2002, *Neuron*, **34**, 13.

164. Mayberg, H. S. 1997, *Neuroreport*, **8**, 1057.

165. Mayberg, H. S. 2002, *Semin. Clin. Neuropsychiatry*, **7**, 255.

166. Bremner, J. D., Vythilingam, M., Ng, C. K., et al. 2003, *JAMA*, **289**, 3125.

167. Kugaya, A. and Sanacora, G. 2005, *CNS Spectr.*, **10**, 808.

168. Yildiz-Yesiloglu, A. and Ankerst, D. P. 2006, *Psychiatry Res.*, **147**, 1.

169. Ende, G., Braus, D. F., Walter, S., Weber-Fahr, W., and Henn, F. A. 2000, *Arch. Gen. Psychiatry*, **57**, 937.

170. Michael, N., Erfurth, A., Ohrmann, P., et al. 2003, *Psychopharmacology (Berl)*, **168**, 344.

171. Zarate, C. A., Jr., Singh, J. B., Carlson, P. J., et al. 2006, *Arch. Gen. Psychiatry*, **63**, 856.

172. Chang, L., Cloak, C. C., and Ernst, T. 2003, *J. Clin. Psychiatry*, **64** Suppl 3, 7.

173. Sanacora, G., Mason, G. F., Rothman, D. L., et al. 1999, *Arch. Gen. Psychiatry*, **56**, 1043.

174. Sanacora, G., Mason, G. F., Rothman, D. L., and Krystal, J. H. 2002, *Am. J. Psychiatry*, **159**, 663.

175. Sanacora, G., Mason, G. F., Rothman, D. L., et al. 2003, *Am. J. Psychiatry*, **160**, 577.

176. Bhagwagar, Z., Wylezinska, M., Jezzard, P., et al. 2008, *Int. J. Neuropsychopharmacol.*, **11**, 255.

177. Cryan, J. F. and Kaupmann, K. 2005, *Trends Pharmacol. Sci.*, **26**, 36.

178. Nestler, E. J. and Carlezon, W. A., Jr. 2006, *Biol. Psychiatry*, **59**, 1151.

179. Volkow, N. D., Chang, L., Wang, G. J., et al. 2001, *Am. J. Psychiatry*, **158**, 2015.

180. Hyder, F. 2009, *Methods Mol. Biol.*, **489**, 3.

181. Shah, Y. B., Haynes, L., Prior, M. J., Marsden, C. A., Morris, P. G., and Chapman, V. 2005, *Psychopharmacology (Berl)*, **180**, 761.

182. Littlewood, C. L., Jones, N., O'Neill, M. J., Mitchell, S. N., Tricklebank, M., and Williams, S. C. 2006, *Psychopharmacology (Berl)*, **186**, 64.

183. Gozzi, A., Large, C. H., Schwarz, A., Bertani, S., Crestan, V., and Bifone, A. 2008, *Neuropsychopharmacology*, **33**, 1690.

184. Langley Langley, T. A., O'Neill, M. J., Mitchell, S., Jones, N., Williams, S. C. 2007, Society for Neuroscience Online, Program No. 501.9.

185. Czeh, B., Michaelis, T., Watanabe, T., et al. 2001, *Proc. Natl Acad. Sci. USA*, **98**, 12796.

186. Michael-Titus, A. T., Albert, M., Michael, G. J., et al. 2008, *Eur. J. Pharmacol.*, **598**, 43.

187. Sartorius, A., Vollmayr, B., Neumann-Haefelin, C., Ende, G., Hoehn, M., and Henn, F. A. 2003, *Neuroreport*, **14**, 2199.

188. Sartorius, A., Mahlstedt, M. M., Vollmayr, B., Henn, F. A., and Ende, G. 2007, *Neuroreport*, **18**, 1469.

189. Artigas, F. and Adell, A. 2007, *Handbook of Microdialysis*, New York, Academic Press, 527.

190. Millan, M. J. 2007, *Handbook of Microdialysis*, New York, Academic Press, 485.

191. Pomerleau, F., Day, B. K., Huettl, P., Burmeister, J. J., and Gerhardt, G. A. 2003, *Ann. NY Acad. Sci.*, **1003**, 454.

192. van der Stelt, H. M., Breuer, M. E., Olivier, B., and Westenberg, H. G. 2005, *Biol. Psychiatry*, **57**, 1061.

193. Gronli, J., Fiske, E., Murison, R., et al. 2007, *Behav. Brain Res.*, **181**, 42.

194. Di Chiara, G., Loddo, P., and Tanda, G. 1999, *Biol. Psychiatry*, **46**, 1624.

195. Kalivas, P. W. and Volkow, N. D. 2005, *Am. J. Psychiatry*, **162**, 1403.

196. Kirby, L. G. and Lucki, I. 1997, *J. Pharmacol. Exp. Ther.*, **282**, 967.

197. Page, M. E., Brown, K., and Lucki, I. 2003, *Psychopharmacology (Berl)*, **165**, 194.

198. Linthorst, A. C., Flachskamm, C., and Reul, J. M. 2008, *Stress*, **11**, 88.

199. de Groote, L. and Linthorst, A. C. 2007, *Neuroscience*, **148**, 794.

Chapter

4 Translational research in mood disorders: using imaging technologies in biomarker research

Jul Lea Shamy, Adam M. Brickman, Chris D. Griesemer, Anna Parachikova, and Mark Day

Abstract

Dramatic scientific and technological advances in the field of drug discovery have been made over the past decade, without a corresponding improvement in the success rate of compounds in clinical development. In response, translational research was developed as a research discipline with the aim of improving the correspondence between preclinical and clinical success of therapeutic treatments by identifying novel disease biomarkers, drug targets, and mechanisms of action for compounds of interest. Functional magnetic resonance imaging (fMRI) and positron emission tomography (PET) have been widely used to reveal the neurobiological underpinnings of human cognition and emotion. The knowledge gained from such studies is currently being employed in the clinical setting to better diagnose and develop treatments for mood disorders. Many of the imaging techniques established in humans are now feasible in animal models (rodents and non-human primates), allowing closer alignment of imaging biomarkers across species and improved congruency between the laboratory and clinical setting. In this review, we explore the use of neuroimaging biomarkers as a translational technique to pave the way to improved clinical success through greater psychiatric disease understanding.

Introduction

Mood disorders, including major depressive disorder (MDD) and the bipolar disorders (BD) are among the leading causes of disability for Americans between the ages of 15 and 44 years [1]. As defined by the DSM-IV-TR, MDD is characterized by one or more major depressive episodes, often with additional symptoms of anhedonia, irritability, difficulty concentrating, and disturbances of sleep and eating. BD is characterized by both the symptoms of MDD and at least one manic episode as defined by heightened mood, exaggerated sense of self-worth, aggression, delusions, and hallucinations [2]. In any given year, MDD and BD affect approximately 14.8 and 5.7 million Americans, respectively [1,3,4].

Understanding the mechanisms of these abnormalities of emotion processing may prove to be helpful in the diagnosis, treatment, and prevention of mood disorders. Generally, MDD and BD are considered "functional" disorders associated with abnormal perception of, reaction to, and memory processing of emotional stimuli – as opposed to one with clearly

Next Generation Antidepressants: Moving Beyond Monoamines to Discover Novel Treatment Strategies for Mood Disorders, ed. Chad E. Beyer and Stephen M. Stahl. Published by Cambridge University Press.
© Cambridge University Press 2010.

defined neuropathology, such as the dopaminergic cell loss observed in Parkinson's disease. As such, non-invasive in-vivo neuroimaging techniques have an important role in furthering our understanding of these disorders and in the development of novel treatments [5–8]. In this chapter, we will discuss the use of functional neuroimaging biomarkers as applied in translational research and drug discovery for the treatment of mood disorders, with a focus on MDD and depressive aspects of BD.

Translational research in drug discovery and development

Translational research, as applied in the pharmaceutical industry, is a research discipline aimed at improving the clinical success of drug discovery and development. As the current success rate of bringing a drug from discovery to market is only about 8% and requires a process of 10–15 years at an average cost of just under $1 billion US [9], this discipline has become a high priority in both the private and academic health sectors. Translational research aims to establish surrogate biomarkers, defined as substances or parameters that can be monitored objectively and reliably reproduced to predict drug effect or outcome [10,11]. Translational approaches are not a substitute for traditional endpoints in clinical trials, but instead are intended to reduce the financial and safety risks associated with large, lengthy, and expensive registration trials [12–14].

Historically, drugs were introduced to humans through empiricism and serendipitous exposure to plant or animal products. Similarly, the original treatments for MDD, the monoamine oxidase inhibitor (MAOI) iproniazid, and the norepinephrine reuptake inhibitor imipramine, were selected based on psychiatric side effects of drugs intended for other clinical purposes [15]. In contrast, drug discovery today is driven primarily by the scientific method, which has enabled the identification of biologically active substances. Our scientific knowledge and technological advances have provided the foundation and capabilities to synthetically alter natural substances to improve potency, duration of action and exposure, or to mitigate undesirable side effects [16].

Of the pharmaceutical therapeutics for MDD currently on the market, 40% of patients that respond to treatment do not show improvement on the first drug prescribed, and about 30% of all patients with MDD do not respond to any of the available drugs (e.g. [17]). In attempts to achieve a therapeutic outcome, individuals who are resistant to treatment are typically managed pharmacologically by switching, increasing, or combining multiple drugs [18,19]. The long lag time between the initiation of antidepressant treatment and remission of symptoms further delays the remission of symptoms in those that do respond to the second- or third-tier drug treatments. It is possible that the lack of response to treatment may be due to a failure to initiate the intended biological response to the medication. Further, depressive symptomology caused by different etiologies may require different treatments. In this context, the use of neuroimaging techniques complements traditional assays of drug metabolism to identify predictors of treatment response and to select those patients most likely to benefit from alternative therapies available through clinical trials. Moreover, the ability to longitudinally evaluate drug effects permits the evaluation of drug treatments acutely and delayed activity of the drug over the lag period observed in both clinical and preclinical animal models.

Preclinical animal models for translational research

The most commonly used preclinical animal model in translational studies is the rodent, due to the short lifespan and disease progression time, well-defined health status with in-bred strains, and a large body of lesion and electrophysiological data upon which to make inferences on the neurobiological basis of affective bias and cognitive impairment. Moreover, mice provide a model that requires comparatively minimal amounts of compound to achieve therapeutic dosing levels. Non-human primates were also developed as translational models largely due to their neuroanatomical, behavioral, and phylogenetic proximity to humans [20]. Non-human primates are used for cognitive and social/affective studies employing social, stimulus, and restraint stressors in conjunction with behavioral tasks designed to mimic clinical tests and to evaluate genetic predisposition [21–24]. Unlike humans, however, they are typically drug-naive, but as they are very valuable, they are often used for more than one study, requiring long washout periods. Still, the non-human primate is well-suited for modeling mood disorders because, similar to humans, they have complex social interactions and social hierarchies. In contrast to humans, the rearing environment of non-human primates can be tightly controlled, which enables the evaluation of interactions between genetic predisposition (nature) and environmental factors (nurture) (for a review, see [25]).

As applied in drug discovery and development, animal models of mood disorders are designed to (1) provide a behavioral model in which to screen potential antidepressant treatments, and/or (2) provide a model with disease biomarkers similar to those used in humans that can be monitored for improvement under antidepressant treatments (for a review see [26]). Most of the currently available animal models of mood disorders are of the former type, such as the forced swim test [27] and learned helplessness test [28] in rodents. These types of drug screens only establish that an antidepressant or non-antidepressant compound, respectively, does or does not reliably affect the behavior of an animal on the task [26]. These are financially advantageous drug screens at early stages of drug discovery as they tend to be sensitive to the acute effects of drug treatment, thereby only requiring limited amounts of drug, time, and resources. As such, these drug screening methods are invaluable for the identification of novel compounds in drug classes already identified as antidepressants. Still, it is the latter type of animal model that is likely to be the key to the success of preclinical drug discovery efforts intended to identify new drug targets with therapeutic potential for mood disorders. To do this, it is necessary to establish models with the same measureable biomarkers as those that occur in the clinical presentation of mood disorders, with similar etiology as the disorder and that can be improved with treatment (e.g. face, construct, and predictive validity). Improved correspondence of basic research and clinical outcome can be achieved by utilizing technologies that can be applied in both animal models and human patients, such as neuroimaging. Through the use of imaging techniques in conjunction with cognitive, affective, and biological biomarkers, it is possible to select or induce preclinical animal models with similarly affected pathways and evaluate the acute and longitudinal effects of therapeutics on these systems.

Translational neuroimaging

In-vivo imaging techniques have the potential to be a powerful, sensitive, and repeatable tool in our translational medicine armamentarium. The applications of neuroimaging in the process of drug discovery and development have been the topic of many supportive and critical reviews in the past few years [5–7,29,30]. The ability to longitudinally evaluate in-vivo measures of disease progression and therapeutic effects of drug treatments is particularly valuable to drug discovery efforts in mood disorders, as the therapeutic effects of antidepressants tend to have a lag of several weeks of administration until clinical efficacy.

Table 4.1 Comparisons of PET and fMRI techniques

Positron emission tomography (PET)	Functional magnetic resonance imaging (fMRI-BOLD)
Measure	Measure
Metabolism: direct: binding of 18FDG PET	Metabolism: indirect via hemodynamic response
Blood flow: 18FDG PET	Blood flow: Hemodynamic response
Ligand binding: direct: conguate 18FDG or 11C or ligand	Ligand binding: indirect: additional downstream & postsynaptic effects
Advantages	Advantages
In-vivo binding assays advantageous over autoradiography	Non-invasive (no injection needed)
Binding-specific site	High spatial resolution
Direct biomarker of receptor-specific actions	Better temporal resolution than PET
Possible to quantify binding	Obtain multiple types of scans in one session (i.e. structure and function)
Limitations	Limitations
Ligand preparation requires radiochemistry lab	Cannot be used for ligand binding
Requires access or proximity to cyclotron, radiochemistry lab	Sensitive to motion artifacts
Radiation exposure limits number of scans per subject	Some subjects cannot tolerate confinement in magnet
Limited temporal resolution	Some areas are difficult to image (e.g. near sinuses)

PET images of humans were first generated in the early 1970s, nearly a decade before their MRI counterparts. In-depth discussion of the physics and methodology have been described in detail elsewhere (e.g. microPET [31], clinical PET [32]). Briefly, PET produces three-dimensional images reflecting the distribution of radioactively labeled molecules, peptides, antibodies, and/or nanoparticles in the body. An image is created as the radioactive isotope "tag" decays, releasing a positron. This particle quickly collides with an electron in the surrounding matter, and high-energy gamma rays called annihilation photons are produced, emanating from the site in 180° opposing directions and are detected with scintillation material attached to surrounding ring of detectors (as discussed by [33]). Downstream computers employ an array of algorithms to reconstruct a three-dimensional image showing the distribution of all recorded decay events [31]. The technique is sensitive enough to measure picomolar concentrations of labeled biomolecules and therefore it is of great use in the evaluation of the effects of drugs and disease progression on regional metabolism and receptor function.

In drug discovery, positron emission tomography or PET is the primary imaging method employed to measure efficacy, target–compound interaction, and pharmacodynamic biomarkers (for a review see [34]). Fluorine-18-labeled deoxyglucose, also known as FDG, is the conventional "gold standard" method in which to evaluate activity in the brain via glucose consumption. However, the limited spatial (>1 mm preclinical, >2 mm clinical) and temporal resolution (minutes) have made functional magnetic resonance imaging (fMRI) techniques (described later) more appealing for real-time evaluations of emotional and cognitive responses. For further comparisons, see Table 4.1.

MRI is primarily employed for its revelation of gross brain structure and disease; however, for the evaluation of brain function, fMRI is increasingly used in clinical and preclinical settings [35]. fMRI has been used since the 1990s to investigate the wide array of brain activity under a plethora of different behavioral and pharmacological testing conditions. fMRI is often considered almost synonymous with blood oxygen level-dependent (BOLD) imaging; however, the latter is merely one particular measurement in an arsenal of techniques available in fMRI. BOLD imaging utilizes local deoxyhemoglobin as an endogenous contrast agent, relying upon the paramagnetic property of the ferrous iron on the heme of deoxyhemoglobin [35,36]. As the paramagnetic state leads to decreased MRI signal, one might expect to be seeking out a decrease in intensity in order to map an increase in function. However, this effect is more than counterbalanced by associated local increase in cerebral blood flow (CBF) and blood volume (CBV), leading to relative signal increase when compared with baseline maps of the subject's brain. As novel fMRI measurements abound, there has been considerable critical examination of the correlated physiological underpinnings of fMRI signal, especially regarding BOLD (see [37,38]). Although BOLD imaging is still adolescent in its clinical applications, its relatively recent explosion as a research tool has quickly led it to be used as a neurosurgical preparation tool, for investigation of functional abnormalities associated with disease, and as an indicator of pharmacologically derived improvements in brain function [39].

fMRI has been increasingly implemented to better characterize disorders such as depression and bipolar disorder, and as a result, new biomarkers related to functional connectivity for subcategorization have come about (see [40], for example). Recent work in this arena has included basic characterization, such as comparing resting functional patterns in control subjects versus those classified as having major depression [41], as well as investigation of more specific hypotheses, such as the relationship between deficit in working memory and the lack of resolution of neurocognitive deficits following recovery from bipolar disorder [42].

An application of fMRI with particular interest for drug discovery and development is the use of these techniques to evaluate the effect of drugs on the modulation of neural activity, called pharmacological MRI (phMRI; [43,44]). This has the potential to (1) identify the mechanism of action of novel compounds by training a classifier to identify therapeutics for compounds to a reference set (as discussed in [5]), and (2) identify novel therapeutics by evaluating the effects of compounds on disease biomarkers [39]. Although this field is in the early stages of development, it already has demonstrated important contributions to our understanding of the serotonergic system [45,46], some of which will be discussed in the following sections.

These PET and fMRI techniques have been developed to differing degrees for use in preclinical animal models. Although PET scans are typically acquired in the anesthetized animal, the labeled compound is injected while the animal is still awake to minimize the effects of the anesthesia. Although anesthesia is still primarily used in fMRI studies in animal models, imaging methods in conscious rodents and non-human primates have been developed [47] by habituating the animals to the confinement and noise of the scanner prior to the acquisition of the images.

While fMRI provides high spatiotemporal resolution compared to PET, the specificity of the response is limited by the spacing of the capillaries in the brain (>50 μm) and the inability to distinguish activity originating from discrete cell populations (e.g. excitatory vs. inhibitory). Moreover, while it is used to infer, for example, cognition, which is not directly observable, fMRI employs hemodynamic modalities to ascertain spatiotemporal information so it is also employing a surrogate marker of activity to assess mass action. Still, MRI has been described as the most important advancement in imaging since the introduction of the X-ray [37], in large part due to the ability of fMRI to evaluate information processing across the entire brain.

Applications of neuroimaging to biomarker research

In order to establish quantifiable parameters to reliably predict drug effect or outcome, translational research employs biomarkers, also called endophenotypes [48]. These biomarkers aid in (1) identification of disease biomarkers and clinical endpoints, (2) the relevance of the drug target to human disease, (3) the drug interaction with the target, (4) the consequences of target modulation by the drug (pharmacodynamics) in respect to efficacy and safety, and (5) patient selection for the best medical outcome (utilitarian definition by Feuerstein et al. [14]). Neuroimaging techniques can be applied to all of these biomarker categories in drug discovery and development efforts for novel treatments for mood disorders.

Disease biomarkers

Disease biomarkers are measures that covary with disease progression and severity, and thereby act as quantifiable endpoints to evaluate the success of therapeutic compounds [10,49–53]. Whereas in oncology disease markers such as tumor growth and suppression can be visually confirmed with imaging technologies, the hallmarks of mood disorders – emotional and cognitive dysfunction – are not directly observable. In other words, effective emotional and cognitive processing must be inferred from behavior or test results, as opposed to direct observation [54]. Imaging technologies offer a window to investigate the brain regions and circuits that are engaged during emotional or cognitive processing.

Negative bias

Negative bias is one of the most consistently reported findings in depressed individuals and is defined as the tendency to focus on negative stimuli (faces, words, memories, and scenes) and identify neutral stimuli as negative as opposed to positive or neutral (for a review, see [55,56]). The neural response in the brain underlying this negative bias is studied with the use of fMRI activation paradigms. These paradigms typically involve the evaluation of brain activity during the presentation, recall, or classification of words, pictures, or faces with emotional valence compared to neutral stimuli or resting conditions [57]. The brain regions involved in these behavioral tests typically include various combinations of the fusiform gyrus, superior temporal sulcus, amygdala, anterior insula, orbitofrontal cortex, ventral striatum, the anterior cingulate cortex and the prefrontal cortex [58–60].

In depressed patients compared to healthy control subjects, the primary imaging biomarker of negative bias is relatively increased activation in the amygdala in response to fearful faces. The amygdala response compared to baseline is relatively stable across testing sessions [61], and can be ameliorated with eight weeks of treatment with fluoxetine hydrochloride [62]. The ability to measure this biomarker reliably across multiple testing sessions is particularly important for evaluating compounds that have a lag time of two weeks or more to see clinical efficacy, as is the case with many antidepressant compounds.

In addition to measurement of regional changes in activity of the amygdala, several lines of evidence support the use of network "connectivity" models for evaluation of disease mechanisms and treatment effects. In depressed patients, negative bias is related to increased activation in the amygdala and greater functional connectivity with the hippocampus and striatum [63], perhaps contributing to the inability of patients with depression to ignore emotional cues [60,64]. Further, in response to negative pictures, patients with MDD showed coordinated increases of activation in the amygdala, pallidostriatum, insula, anterior cingulate cortex, and anteromedial prefrontal cortex and decreased connectivity between the anterior cingulate and other limbic regions, perhaps reflecting reduced functional connectivity and feedback between certain cortical and limbic brain structures resulting in maladaptive responses to neutral stimuli [65]. Moreover, an eight-week therapeutic regimen of fluoxetine hydrochloride can increase coupling between the cortical–limbic systems (amygdala, frontal and cingulate cortex, striatum, and thalamus [66]).

Cognitive deficits

Cognitive or neuropsychological functioning, which comprises domains such as attention, learning and memory, visuospatial functioning, language abilities, processing speed, and executive functioning, is another potential biomarker or endophenotype in the clinical syndrome of depression [54,55]. Clinical and experimental cognitive probes that are used to stimulate frontal cortex activity, such as the Wisconsin Card Sorting Test (WCST; [19]) and n-back tasks [67], are very amenable to fMRI study designs and are frequently used to evaluate frontal dysfunction in psychiatric disorders. In the WCST, subjects are required to match a sample card with one of four displayed cards according to color, number, or shape. The sorting rule is not told to the patient and the individual must find the rule that governs correct matching. After an unpredictable number of trials, the rule is changed and the participant must learn the new rule. This classic test of executive function measures flexibility in thinking, the capacity to form abstract concepts, and the ability to shift or maintain attentional set. In the n-back task, participants are presented with a series of numbers or letters and asked to indicate whether the current stimulus matches the stimulus n trials earlier. For example, in a "2-back" task, the following sequence of stimuli may be presented and the subject would have to respond affirmatively to all those in bold:

W R B C **B** S C C Q R **Q** K R **K** C Q W R R K

Using such tasks, authors have noted for decades that mood disorders, such as MDD, are associated with neuropsychological deficits in addition to the primary mood disturbance that defines the disorder [68]. The patterns of neuropsychological deficits among patients with MDD usually comprise mild to moderate deficits in effortful learning and memory retrieval, as well as psychomotor speed, and the so-called "executive functioning" [69–71]. From a functional neuroanatomy perspective, we typically consider learning and memory to be supported by the hippocampus and related structures, suggesting that MDD comprises functional deficiencies in these regions. However, closer examination of the behavioral pattern of neuropsychological performance among patients with MDD would suggest that memory deficits are not "amnestic" per se, but rather are the result of effortful processing, sustained attention, and retrieval deficits. In fact, when patients with MDD are given retrieval cues or forced-choice recognition paradigms, their memory performance is often commensurate with unaffected controls. There is, thus, general consensus that the neuropsychological pattern of deficits seen in MDD can be categorized neuroanatomically as "frontal" or "frontal–subcortical." It is important to note that while cognitive dysfunction and altered prefrontal activity are features of mood disorders, they are less severe than that reported in schizophrenia or Alzheimer's disease. Further, selective serotonin reuptake inhibitors (SSRI) pharmacotherapy may increase impairment of cognitive and psychomotor function [72,73].

Preclinical models of affective and cognitive disturbances

Although social interactions, fear reactions, and cognitive processes can be evaluated in both rodents and non-human primate models, it is possible to more directly translate these behavioral tests from the clinic to preclinical setting to evaluate drug efficacy on negative bias and cognitive impairments. For over 60 years, cognitive impairments have been evaluated in non-human primates, originally using the Wisconsin General Testing Apparatus (WGTA [74]) and more recently with automated touch-screen systems, such as Cambridge Neuropsychological Test Automated Battery (CANTAB), that enable more complex testing and higher throughput. Although these techniques are not typically used in evaluation of non-human primate models of depression, there is a high degree of predictability of the clinical effectiveness of cognition-enhancing drugs in humans supporting the evaluation of cognitive impairments and treatments in non-human primate models of depression [75]. PET tracers are often injected prior to a behavioral test or video of stimuli to measure the uptake of the tracer and evaluate the functional consequence of the drug on the functional activity of relevant brain regions. Alternatively, in the context of neural bias, a translational model with direct clinical relevance could be developed, for example, by screening the monkeys for depressive symptoms followed by an fMRI activation paradigm displaying monkey faces and evaluating the response of the amgydala and emotional circuitry in the control versus depressed monkeys (e.g. Hoffman et al. [76]).

The validity of using animal models to evaluate cortical contribution to cognitive and affective processing has been brought into question by some researchers due to the fact that the frontal cortex is relatively smaller in non-human primates than in humans. While monkeys have a modest-sized dorsolateral prefrontal cortex, rodents do not have a discrete area that corresponds to this brain region [77]. Still, monkeys do have a dorsolateral prefrontal cortex, and both rodents and monkeys have thalamic connectivity with orbital and medial frontal regions similar to those primarily associated with processing of emotional information in humans. Indeed, much of the anatomical circuitry involved in emotional perception and processing was first documented in non-human primates using anatomical tracers and lesions and later confirmed using neuroimaging techniques in humans. Taken together, whereas the rodent may have limitations for direct translation of the negative bias and executive dysfunctions mediated by the dorsolateral prefrontal cortex, the non-human primate is well-suited as a preclinical animal model in which to evaluate these biomarkers.

Target validation biomarkers

Target validation biomarkers provide scientific evidence that a segment of DNA, RNA, or a protein molecule is directly involved in a human disease and that it is a suitable target for the development of a new therapeutic drug. Drug discovery formerly focused on only a few known therapeutic targets, but the completion of the human genome project in the year 2000 resulted in the availability of thousands of potential drug targets. Neuroimaging has been employed in conjunction with many target validation techniques including sense reversal (e.g. gene knockouts, antisense technology, and RNA interference [78,79]), proteomics (e.g. manipulating the activity of the potential target protein itself), and pharmacogenomics (e.g. evaluation of individual variations in the candidate gene, single nucleotide polymorphisms (SNPs), or gene expression [80] and transgenic animal models (e.g. genes are deleted or disrupted to halt their expression) (for review see [81,82]).

Phamacogenomics

Pharmacogenomics is defined as the application of genomic technologies including gene sequencing, statistical genetics, and analysis of gene expression for drug development [30]. In mood disorders, there can be both differing and/or overlapping patterns of cognitive dysfunction, affective bias, morphological and functional neuropathology, and familial risk [83]. One possibility for such variability of results is that genetic variations of particular alleles could be partially responsible for the concordance and discordance within the disorders [84]. There are several identified susceptibility genes including the polymorphism of the serotonin transporter gene (5-HTT). There is evidence that, compared to those homozygous for the long allele (ll), the carriers of a short (s) allele of the 5-HTT promoter polymorphism is related to an increased risk for depressive symptoms in humans [85–87] (but see [88]) and anxiety behaviors in non-human primates (e.g. [25,89–91]).

fMRI studies show healthy individuals and depressed patients with the short allele as compared to the long allele demonstrate a robust increase in amygdala response to threat-related facial expressions and other aversive emotional stimuli and a decrease in functional connectivity between the ventral anterior cingulate cortex (vACC) and the amygdala [92–94]. During fear and happy face processing, patients with BD have significantly lower vACC activation compared to healthy controls, and across both groups, short alelle carriers have lower activation than those individuals with homozygous long alleles, such that BD short allele carriers exhibit the greatest magnitude of vACC dysfunction. Notably, while this polymorphism may affect expression of some aspects of the serotonergic network (e.g. 5-HT1A receptors; [95]), there does not appear to be a significant relationship between s-allele carrier status and in-vivo 5-HTT binding as measured by PET imaging in either humans or non-human primates (measured by [^{11}C]DASB; [96–98]).

Clearly, there are many other polymorphisms in various genes to be considered, and it is likely that pharmacological efficacy in mood disorders will depend on the sum of small effects from multiple genes and interactions between them [96]. As this is a developing field, care must be taken to avoid overstating the connections between individual genes and complex symptomology (see [99]). Still, there is evidence to support imaging genetics as a robust and informative method in which to evaluate genetic variations on brain structure, function, and development of psychiatric disease [47].

Transgenic mice

Although thousands of genetically manipulated animals have been generated for target validation in neurodegenerative disorders, there are comparatively few in psychiatric disorders, including mood disorders. Transgenic models developed for depression including those with variations in 5-HTT (e.g. SERT; [100,101]) and BD (e.g. WFS1 [84] and Disc1 [103]) may be uninformative to the study of mood disorders. The evaluation of these lines may provide insight about the role of the target in human diseases, and the target's potential for manipulation and exploitation in drug discovery and development. For example, alterations of behavioral measures and functional connectivity of the reward circuit both occur in the SERT knockout mouse [84]. The serotonin transporter (SERT) affects multiple aspects of the monoaminergic system by modulating the entire serotonergic system and influencing the dopaminergic and norepinephrinergic systems. When manganese was injected into the frontal cortex of SERT knockout mice, the active circuitry originating in the prefrontal cortex in the SERT knockout was altered, shifting activity from frontal to posterior regions including the substantia nigra, ventral tegmental area, and Raphé nuclei. It is worth noting that even though this difference had little effect on metabolite levels or connectivity as measured by magnetic resonance spectroscopy (MRS) and diffusion tensor imaging, it supports the value of in-vivo functional techniques as a part of target validation of transgenic mouse models of mood disorders.

Target–compound interaction and pharmacokinetic/pharmacodynamic biomarkers

Target–compound interaction biomarkers provide evidence of the physical–chemical interaction of the drug with its intended target. PET imaging is used in drug development by radiolabeling drugs with radioisotopes such as carbon-11 (^{11}C) or fluorine-18 (^{18}F) for the evaluation of target binding, residency time, specific site of interaction, and the physical or chemical consequences to the target induced by the compound. By establishing the relationship between drug exposure (dose or plasma concentration) and renal output, it is possible to select appropriate doses for therapeutic doses and unsafe doses prior to clinical trials.

Like all in-vivo imaging studies, investigations using PET are thoughtfully designed to not significantly affect the physiology under investigation. There are a couple of particular advantages to PET. First, the radioactive label, attached directly or even through use of a chelating agent, is small as compared with fluorescent or MRI reporter groups, minimizing influence on the properties of the target-specific drug [104]. Additionally, only a small amount of radioactive-labeled compound is injected (i.e. the tracer principle [105,106]). Besides its general scientific merit, this design principle has a direct effect on the way novel diagnostic imaging agents are brought to clinical trials. The Food and Drug Administration regulates novel imaging probes in a manner parallel to novel pharmaceuticals. However, recognition of the small amounts of probe needed for PET tracers has created a less cumbersome exploratory version of the Investigational New Drug requirements, the eIND, which permits more expedient clinical trials [107].

Pharmacokinetic and pharmacodynamic biomarkers predict the distribution, metabolism, excretion, receptor binding, postreceptor effects, and chemical interactions of a drug. Pharmacokinetic information is often obtained using high-performance liquid chromatography (HPLC) or mass spectroscopy to measure drug concentration at multiple time points in plasma or urine samples. However, in many cases, the kinetics (e.g. concentration, magnitude of peak, and time course) of a drug in the brain differs from that in the plasma. By using in-vivo imaging, it is possible to establish the relationship between plasma concentration and target occupancy, tissue distribution and metabolism of the drug to aid in the interpretation of therapeutic relevance of plasma PK/PD measures.

PET imaging is the standard imaging method employed for in-vivo PK/PD studies as it enables the monitoring of the absolute radioactivity concentrations in tissues pixel-by-pixel. In addition to the target–compound interactions, these imaging biomarkers can be used to evaluate a novel compound for which there is yet no tracer. In this case, the drug effect can be evaluated indirectly by quantifying the displacement of the ligand in the target system (see [105] for review).

A major hurdle in designing drugs directed at the brain is that hydrophilic compounds are unable to cross the blood–brain barrier (BBB), and of those small molecules that do cross the BBB, 98% do not cross in sufficient amounts [105,108]. Among other constraints, to enter the CNS in the presence of an intact BBB, the compound must be sufficiently liposoluble and weigh less than 180 Daltons ([109]). Still, compounds that meet these requirements may not enter the brain due to other factors, including active efflux pumps, degree of ionization, and plasma protein binding. These difficulties have traditionally been circumvented using PET ligands, due to their aforementioned small size.

By using radiolabeled receptor ligands, it is possible to evaluate the biodistribution of a compound, including the density of receptors in a medication-free state, or to evaluate the amount of unblocked receptors in a medication-treated state. The most widely accepted method of imaging the 5-HT1A serotonin receptors is through carbon-11-labeled ligand, [^{11}C]DASB. This tracer offers both high selectivity and a favorable ratio of specific binding relative to free and non-specific binding enabling a reliable quantitation of the 5-HTT binding potential (reviewed by [108]). As visualized with this ligand, patients with MDD and dysphoria have elevated 5-HTT binding in relevant brain regions. Further, SSRI administration at optimal therapeutic doses result in 80% 5-HTT receptor occupancy compared to placebo [110]. Other serotonergic ligands include [^{11}C]WAY-100635 which binds to both 5-HT1A [110] and D2 receptors and [^{18}F]-altanserin for 5-HT2A receptor [111].

In addition, MRS can be used to evaluate changes in the concentration of both the parent drug and of the metabolites. Magnetic resonance spectroscopy, the underlying principle of MRI, can be used to detect the distribution of nuclei with particular spin properties. Whereas MRI focuses on the spin signals generated by protons in water and fat, MRS can image a variety of nuclei. As the technique follows the nuclear signal, it can be used to evaluate changes in the concentration of both the parent drug and of the metabolites in the brain. This is of particular value for testing drugs for mood disorders where proton [^{1}H] spectroscopy can assess glutamate (excitatory) and GABA (inhibitory) amino acids [112]. Brain metabolite concentrations of lithium [^{7}Li] and drugs with a fluorine atom [^{19}F] can be evaluated using MRS (e.g. fluoxetine, fluvoxamine, and paroxetine) [113]. For visualization of metabolites, MRS requires higher concentrations of drug than PET imaging; however, this technique enables longitudinal assessments because ionizing radiation is not required nor are the blood draws required for PK information in PET imaging needed. For example, ^{19}F MRS has been used to evaluate the pharmacokinetics of R-fluoxetine and racemic fluoxetine and identified that a dose of 120 mg/day of R-fluoxetine would be needed to achieve brain levels of active drug comparable to 20 mg/day of racemate [114]. However, based on ECG data, it is unlikely that such a level of R-sfluoxetine should be used. This type of information, when obtained early in the clinical discovery process, can significantly reduce the number of trials needed to define the therapeutic dose range (minimal effective dose/maximal tolerated dose [MED/MTD]) and contribute to more efficient utilization of resources in early drug discovery.

Patient selection and stratification biomarkers

Patient selection and stratification biomarkers provide information on those patients most likely to respond (or not) to the treatment in proof-of-concept (POC) studies or phase II clinical trials. Genetic, pharmacogenomic, and pharmacodynamic measures can be used in conjunction with neuroimaging to stratify patients according to their risk profiles. This approach can potentially enable shorter trials with higher event rates and earlier outcome assessments.

Disease biomarkers

Neuroimaging techniques afford the potential to distinguish patients with affective or cognitive biases that are driven primarily by medial temporal lobe and/or by frontal lobe dysfunction (e.g. episodic memory/affective bias vs. executive function deficits) within a clinical trial. Early PET studies done with [^{18}F]-deoxyglucose showed decreased metabolic activity in prefrontal cortical regions and the amygdala. These findings have been replicated in fMRI studies, and activations in these regions have strong predictive value for response to monoaminergic treatment. Further, there is an apparent dissociation between subregions of the anterior cingulate cortex that predict symptom severity versus those that predict treatment response [115] and antidepressant treatment increases metabolic rate in the dorso lateral prefrontal cortex concomitant with symptom remissions. In contrast to the depressed state, patients in BD I mania demonstrate reduced levels of activity in the amygdala and subgenual cingulate in response to sad facial expressions. Further, correct classification of depressed subjects has been achieved with 86% accuracy during implicit memory processing of sad faces and a more modest accuracy of classification during a working memory task. These studies offer the possibility of using fMRI measures as a patient selection biomarker in early clinical studies. Applied in early clinical studies, one can potentially turn heterogeneous clinical populations into discrete, focused subgroups in which to answer specific questions and prove focused hypotheses about the target patient population and ultimately increase the probability of seeing an effect with a compound while improving the potential for differentiation from comparators. This in turn can aid patient selection in larger phase III studies.

Pharmacogenomics for patient stratification

Through the use of genomics and pharmacogenomics, genetic markers can be used to select optimal medications and dosages for individual patients thereby improving the efficacy, safety, and probability of the patient to respond to a particular drug. This is true for the two examples discussed in this chapter: 5HTT and brain-derived neurotrophic factor (BDNF). The polymormphism of the 5-HTTLPR has been related to the efficacy and onset of theraupeutic response by SSRI treatments.

Presymptomatic diagnosis using neuroimaging in surrogate populations

A new therapeutic focus is to develop treatments that delay the onset or progression of psychiatric disorders. fMRI biomarkers can be used to identify altered patterns of brain activation in individuals at high risk for developing a psychiatric disorder identified by familial risk or pharamacogenomics, and also by evaluating individuals in surrogate populations, such as those with subclinical dysphoria disorder. Several studies have shown that in individuals with subclinical dysphoria, there are significant changes in fMRI responses in temporal lobe regions using emotional fMRI activation studies following administration of antidepressants. This type of information could be used to improve identification of likely candidates for conversion, to identify the stage of the disease, and/or to assess the therapeutic response. In the future, this class of imaging studies could be used in early drug development to provide evidence of antidepressive or anxiolytic activity and subsequently more traditional POC clinical trials in depressed patients.

Non-monoaminergic

Hypothalamic–pituitary–adrenal axis

In conjunction with environmental stressors and genetic predisposition, the activity of the hypothalamic–pituitary–adrenal (HPA) axis is largely considered to be a major risk factor for the development of depression. The hypothalamus controls the activity of these regions by secreting corticotropic-releasing factor (CRF) and vasopressin (AVP). These in turn signal the pituitary gland to secrete adrenocorticotropic hormone (ACTH), which finally stimulates the adrenal cortex to secrete glucocorticoids (i.e. cortisol). Cortisol then modulates the HPA axis activity by providing inhibitory feedback on the hypothalamus and pituitary gland. Moreover, whereas the amygdala and orbitofrontal cortex may stimulate the HPA axis [116–118], the hippocampus may be more involved in negative feedback of the system [119–121].

Clinical symptoms of dysfunction of the HPA axis in MDD includes basal hypercortiso-lemia at baseline [122], elevated cortisol secretion with the dexamethasone suppression test (DST) [123], and increased adrenocorticotropic hormone (ACTH) and cortisol release in the combined dexamethasone suppression/corticotropin-releasing hormone (CRH) stimulation (DEX/CRH) test [124,125]). In unmedicated subjects with MDD, a heightened cortisol response to the DEX/CRH test was related to hypometabolism in the medial prefrontal cortex and hypermetabolism in hippocampal and parahippocampal regions as measured by [^{18}F] FDG PET. Further, the subset of patients that responded to treatment had enhanced cortisol responsiveness and regional hypermetabolism in the temporal regions that were normalized with pharmacotherapy.

Rodent and non-human primate models have been important to our understanding of the HPA axis and its dysfunction under stress. ACTH administration in rodents was developed as a model of treatment-resistant depression as it effectively blocks the effects of imipramine in the forced swim test without significantly impacting the efficacy of bupropion, an "atypical" antidepressant (i.e. does not affect serotonergic releasse, reuptake, or binding to postsynaptic receptors) [126,127]. Little is currently known about the functional effects of this model in the rodent. However, it is possible that this type of drug screen will be beneficial for early identification of drugs that may progress to non-human primate and preclinical trials to improve likelihood of successful treatment response in individuals under stress and with overactive ACTH production.

In contrast, the effect of psychosocial stressors is a well-studied phenomenon in non-human primates and the body of knowledge about the functional changes following stressful situations is growing. Early life stress was initially evaluated in non-human primates at a primate center breeding facility intended to reduce transmission of tuberculosis by removing from their mothers soon after birth [128–133]. Non-human primate models of the effects of stress can incorporate restraint, human or resident intruder, separation, isolation, or the presence of threatening objects, all of which can increase circulating levels of cortisol. Notably, increased activation in the bed nucleus of the stria terminalis (BNST) in response to intruder threat [134] and behavioral freezing is predictive of increased amygdala reactivity. Additional studies have demonstrated interactions between genetic background and exposure to environmental stressors [25,135,136]. For example, compared to homozygous (ll) monkeys, s-carrier monkeys show an increased activation in the amygdala when relocated in a social colony [137] as measured by [^{18}F] FDG PET. Taken together, as has been suggested, it may be critically important to evaluate environmental stressors when determining the effect of genetic variation on behavioral phenotype and treatment response [25,137–139].

Neurotrophin contribution

As the monoaminergic hypothesis does not provide an adequate explanation for the lag period between initiation of antidepressant treatment and the therapeutic response, it has been hypothesized that monoaminergic drugs act by secondary mechanisms that induces gene transcriptional and translational changes (see [140,141]). These alterations result in increased hippocampal neurogenesis via alterations in cAMP response element-binding protein (CREB) and protein synthesis in neurotrophic pathways, such as BDNF. Neurotrophins are important regulators of neuronal plasticity and BDNF, in particular, plays a key role in synaptic organization dependent on activity, balancing the effects of excitatory (glutamate) and inhibitory (GABA) transmission. Moreover, BDNF-dependent synaptic reorganization includes shaping those neuronal networks important for behavioral adaptations to environmental stimuli.

A polymorphism in the BDNF gene, specifically the substitution from the amino acid valine to methionine (val66met) at chromosome 11p13 in the region that codes for BDNF, has been associated with depression and BD (for review see: [142,143]). This neurotrophin is a therapeutic target for depression and a potential contributor to cognitive dysfunction in mood disorders. The Val allele appears to increase the risk for bipolar illness [144,145], and is associated with rapid cycling between manic and depressive states [146]. As measured by the fMRI BOLD response, healthy individuals who are carriers for the Met allele (val66met) exhibited decreased hippocampal activity during a declarative memory test [147] and also poorer episodic memory [148] than did individuals homozygous for Val. In individuals with bipolar illness, those with Val compared with Met, had better prefrontal function as measured by H-magnetic resonance spectroscopy [149] and WCST performance [150].

In addition to playing a role in the pathophysiology of mood disorders, BDNF exerts effects on the mechanism of action of therapeutic agents. Mood stabilizers and antidepressants increase levels of BDNF in animal models [151,152] as well as in the clinic [153]. The BDNF polymorphism additionally affects antidepressant treatment outcome. Patients with Val/Met exhibit a more favorable response following lithium treatment [154]. Therapeutically, fluvoxamine, milnacipram [155], and fluoxetine [156] were more effective in subjects with Val/Met than either homozygous. In contrast, patients with the Met allele were responsive to the SSRI citalopram [157]. Further, there appears to be an interaction between Val/Val polymorphism of BDNF and s carrier of 5HTTPRL that can predict 70% non-response to lithium [158].

Inflammation

Another key component of MDD neuropathogenesis is the inflammatory system [159]. Depression has been associated with increased peripheral inflammatory markers capable of accessing the CNS resulting in chronic low-grade inflammation [160]. Chronic brain inflammation results in a cascade of detrimental events culminating in neuronal/synaptic dysfunction and eventual death. In MDD, chronic microglial activation leads to the loss of astrocytes, which further upsets the balance of pro- and anti-inflammatory mediators, impairs removal of excitatory amino acid, and culminates in excitotoxicity (e.g. [161,162]). Moreover, administration of pro-inflammatory molecules including interferon-α in humans [163] and monkeys [164], as well as interleukin-1β in rodents [165] have been shown to elicit depressive symptomology. Hence, inhibiting pro-inflammatory cascades may improve depressed mood and increase treatment response to conventional antidepressant medication. Depressed patients with increased inflammatory biomarkers are more likely to exhibit treatment resistance and antidepressant therapy, which has been associated with decreased inflammatory responses [166]. Furthermore, administration of anti-inflammatories in conjunction with antidepressants, such as acetylsalicylic acid with fluoxetine [167] and celecoxib with reboxetine [168], have demonstrated improved therapeutic response in healthy subjects compared with the antidepressant with placebo.

The immunorestrictive role of the BBB creates a challenge for direct evaluation of the inflammatory response in the brain and, as a result, primarily [^{18}FDG]PET and fMRI methodology has been utilized in the functional evaluation of inflammation in depression. Imaging studies in humans have revealed that inflammatory-related fatigue and psychomotor slowing are related to activity changes in the insula [168,169] and substantia nigra [170]. Further, inflammatory-related emotional depressive symptomology is related to increased activity in the subgenual anterior cingulate cortex (sACC) and circulating levels of IL-6 appear to modulate the functional connectivity of the region with the amygdala, medial prefrontal cortex, and various other regions [171]. Dysfunction of the sACC has also been reported in patients with MDD and can be reversed with administration of SSRIs [170]. It is likely that measuring serum levels of inflammation biomarkers (e.g. C-reactive protein [CRP] and cytokines) may aid in the identification of patients likely to show therapeutic response to an antidepressant and anti-inflammatory combination.

Vascular depression

About a decade ago, the term "vascular depression" was introduced to describe a subgroup of elderly MDD patients whose syndrome appeared to be etiologically related to cerebrovascular disease [172]. The concept emerged from the observation that adults with MDD onset in later life had greater degrees of cerebrovascular disease than similarly aged depressed individuals with earlier onset [173]. Several studies demonstrated that older depressed individuals with vascular depression or with evidence of significant cerebrovascular burden have a neuropsychological profile that includes enhanced deficits in executive abilities and processing speed [174,175]. This suggests that the co-existence of mood disturbance, executive dysfunction, and cerebrovascular disease among older adults defines a unique syndrome. There is still some debate about whether existence of this syndrome points to a single etiological factor, as is suggested by the term "subcortical ischemic depression," which attributes pathogenesis to disruption in frontal–subcortical circuitry due to vascular disease, or to multiple etiological factors as suggested by the term "depression–executive dysfunction syndrome," which suggests that the symptoms frequently co-exist but can be attributable to varied pathology (see [176] for discussion). In either case, it is important to note that neuroimaging plays a central role in characterizing the syndrome. Small vessel cerebrovascular disease, which is visualized as punctate or diffuse areas of increased signal intensity, often referred to as "white matter hyperintensities" (WMH), on T2-weighted/fluid attenuated inverse recovery (FLAIR) structural fMRI scans, is common across a number of conditions in aging. Whether WMH severity or burden can be used as a traditional endophenotype or biomarker in depression trials among older adults is up for some debate. None the less, it is clear from the literature that the presence and severity of cerebrovascular disease among older depressed patients, along with executive dysfunction, is predictive of treatment response [177–180].

Placebo effect

In clinical practice, the placebo effect is beneficial as it maximizes the therapeutic potential for the patient; however, in clinical trials, it is desirable to minimize the inclusion of the phenomenon in order to identify the actual effect of the drug (for review see [181]). Expectation of symptom improvement has long been believed to play a critical role in the placebo effect, particularly in psychiatric disorders. Meta-analyses have shown that the mean rates of response in the placebo group in antidepressant trials are 29.7% [182] and have suggested that differences between the drug and placebo groups might be relatively small in patients with MDD due to the placebo response [183,184]. Notably, the placebo effect has been related to disorder-specific effects, including increase in dopamine release in Parkinson's disease and opioid transmission in pain disorders (see [185] for review). Further, other considerations including spontaneous remission, selection of the placebo, and lack of proper blinding of clinical scientists, physicians, patients, and/or caretakers can also contribute to a non-pharmaceutical-related improvement of depressive symptoms.

Although it is unlikely that these factors will be removed entirely from clinical studies, neuroimaging can be used to separate the drug response from the placebo response. For example, responders to 6-week fluoxetine or placebo both demonstrated metabolic increases in several cortical regions (e.g. prefrontal cortex and parietal cortex) with concomitant decreases in the subcortical regions (e.g. parahippocampus and thalamus; [186,187]). In addition, the fluoxetine-treated groups had metabolic alterations in multiple subcortical regions (e.g. brainstem, striatum, hippocampus). It has been suggested that successful treatment of depression is related to bottom-up actions of antidepressants and top-down activity of the placebo [188] and appears to be functionally distinct from treatment response [188]. By employing neuroimaging techniques, it may be possible to better evaluate the pharmacological and therapeutic potential of lead compounds by removal of subjects with this functional profile of the placebo effect [189]. Further, in the clinic, top-down treatments such as Cognitive Behavior Therapy in conjunction with antidepressant treatments may act to shorten the lag time for drug effect by initiating the top-down cortical control of maladaptive self-defeating, cognitive, and affective styles inherent to MDD.

Summary

As discussed in this chapter and previously discussed by Leuchter et al. [189], disease biomarkers can influence early internal decisions in the discovery and development pipeline and also direct evaluation of all other biomarker classes [14]. In preclinical stages, disease biomarkers are used for selection of potential drug targets, proof-of-concept for target–compound engagement, evaluation of pharmacokinetic–pharmacodynamic relationships on efficacy and safety, and financial risk–benefit assessments. In the development stages, they help in investment decisions for critical phase 3 registration studies and labeling. During the clinical trial stages, disease biomarkers can be applied for diagnostic purposes and to individualize treatment by stratifying the patient population to improve the likelihood of response to various treatments.

With the advent of imaging technologies, it is now possible to conduct in vivo evaluations of these biomarkers in "functional" psychiatric disorders, such as MDD. Through the use of this technology, it is possible to evaluate the underlying neurological changes at a systems level and evaluate the therapeutic response to treatment. Indeed, the application of this technology in drug discovery and development is only recently being realized and is likely to become more influential in the coming years.

References

1. Kessler, R. C., et al., The epidemiology of major depressive disorder: results from the National Comorbidity Survey Replication (NCS-R). *JAMA*, 2003. **289**(23): 3095–105.

2. First, B., M. A. Frances, and H. A. Pincus, *DSM-IV-TR Handbook of Differential Diagnosis*. Arlington, VA, American Psychiatric Publishing, 2002: p. 247.

3. Kessler, R. C., et al., Lifetime prevalence and age-of-onset distributions of DSM-IV disorders in the National Comorbidity Survey Replication. *Arch Gen Psychiatry*, 2005. **62**(6): 593–602.

4. Merikangas, K. R., et al., Lifetime and 12-month prevalence of bipolar spectrum disorder in the National Comorbidity Survey replication. *Arch Gen Psychiatry*, 2007. **64**(5): 543–52.

5. Borsook, D., L. Becerra, and R. Hargreaves, A role for fMRI in optimizing CNS drug development. *Nat Rev Drug Discov*, 2006. **5**(5): 411–25.

6. Wise, R. and I. Tracey, The role of fMRI in drug discovery. *J Magn Reson Imaging*, 2006. **23**(6): 862–76.

7. Wong, D. F., J. Tauscher, and G. Gründer, The role of imaging in proof of concept for CNS drug discovery and development. *Neuropsychopharmacology*, 2009. **34**(1): 187–203.

8. Rudin, M., Noninvasive structural, functional, and molecular imaging in drug development. *Curr Opin Chem Biol*, 2009. **13**(3): 360–71.

9. DiMasi, J. A., R. W. Hansen, and H. G. Grabowski, The price of innovation: new estimates of drug development costs. *J Health Econ*, 2003. **22**(2): 151–85.

10. Lesko, L. J. and A. J. Atkinson, Use of biomarkers and surrogate endpoints in drug development and regulatory decision making: criteria, validation, strategies. *Annu Rev Pharmacol Toxicol*, 2001. **41**: 347–66.

11. Boissel, J. P., et al., Surrogate endpoints: a basis for a rational approach. *Eur J Clin Pharmacol*, 1992. 43(3): 235–44.

12. Williams, S. A., et al., A cost-effectiveness approach to the qualification and acceptance of biomarkers. *Nat Rev Drug Discov*, 2006. **5**(11): 897–902.

13. Feuerstein, G. and J. Chavez, Translational medicine for stroke drug discovery: the pharmaceutical industry perspective. *Stroke*, 2008. **40**(3, Supplement 1): S121–25.

14. Feuerstein G. Z., Rutkowski J. L. R., F. S. Walsh, G. L. Stiles, R. R. Ruffolo Jr, The role of translational medicine and biomarker research in drug discovery and development. *Am Drug Discovery*, 2007. **2**(1): 23–28.

15. Stanford, S. C., Depression. In R. A. Webster (Ed.), *Neurotransmitters, Drugs, and Brain Function*. Chichester, John Wiley, 2001: p. 534.

16. Day, M., J. L. Rutkowski, and G. Z. Feuerstein, Translational medicine – a paradigm shift in modern drug discovery and development: the role of biomarkers. *Adv Exp Med Biol*, 2009. **655**: 1–12.

17. Baghai, T. C., H. P. Volz, and H. J. Moller, Drug treatment of depression in the 2000s: An overview of achievements in the last 10 years and future possibilities. *World J Biol Psychiatry*, 2006. 7(4): 198–222.

18. Little, A., Treatment-resistant depression. *Am Fam Physician*, 2009. **80**(2): 167–72.

19. Rosenzweig-Lipson, S., et al., Differentiating antidepressants of the future: efficacy and safety. *Pharmacol Ther*, 2007. **113**(1): 134–53.

20. Capitanio, J. P. and M. E. Emborg, Contributions of non-human primates to neuroscience research. *Lancet*, 2008. **371** (9618): 1126–35.

21. Kinnally, E. L., et al., Effects of early experience and genotype on serotonin transporter regulation in infant rhesus macaques. *Genes Brain Behav*, 2008. **7**(4): 481–86.

22. Shively, C. A., K. Laber-Laird, and R. F. Anton, Behavior and physiology of social stress and depression in female cynomolgus monkeys. *Biol Psychiatry*, 1997. **41**(8): 871–82.

23. Shively, C. A., et al., Social stress, depression, and brain dopamine in female cynomolgus monkeys. *Ann NY Acad Sci*, 1997. **807**: 574–77.

24. Izquierdo, A., et al., Genetic modulation of cognitive flexibility and socioemotional behavior in rhesus monkeys. *Proc Natl Acad Sci USA*, 2007. **104**(35): 14128–33.

25. Barr, C. S., et al., The utility of the non-human primate; model for studying gene by environment interactions in behavioral research. *Genes Brain Behav*, 2003. **2**(6): 336–40.

26. Rupniak, N. M., Animal models of depression: challenges from a drug development perspective. *Behav Pharmacol*, 2003. **14**(5–6): 385–90.

27. Porsolt, R. D., et al., Immobility induced by forced swimming in rats: effects of agents which modify central catecholamine and serotonin activity. *Eur J Pharmacol*, 1979. **57**(2–3): 201–10.

28. Sherman, A. D., J. L. Sacquitne, and F. Petty, Specificity of the learned helplessness model of depression. *Pharmacol Biochem Behav*, 1982. **16**(3): 449–54.

29. Willmann, J., et al., Molecular imaging in drug development. *Nat Rev Drug Discov*, 2008. **7**(7): 591–607.

30. Hargreaves, R. J., The role of molecular imaging in drug discovery and development. *Clin Pharmacol Ther*, 2008. **83**(2): 349–53.

31. Rowland, D. J. and S. R. Cherry, Small-animal preclinical nuclear medicine instrumentation and methodology. *Semin Nucl Med*, 2008. **38**(3): 209–22.

32. Townsend, D. W., Multimodality imaging of structure and function. *Phys Med Biol*, 2008. **53**(4): R1–39.

33. Cherry, S. R., J. A. Sorenson, and M. E. Phelps. *Physics in Nuclear Medicine*, Philadelphia, PA, Saunders, 2003, p. 523.

34. Lee, C. M. and L. Farde, Using positron emission tomography to facilitate CNS drug development. *Trends Pharmacol Sci*, 2006. **27**(6): 310–16.

35. Ogawa, S., et al., Brain magnetic resonance imaging with contrast dependent on blood oxygenation. *Proc Natl Acad Sci USA*, 1990. **87**(24): 9868–72.

36. Ogawa, S., et al., Intrinsic signal changes accompanying sensory stimulation: functional brain mapping with magnetic resonance imaging. *Proc Natl Acad Sci USA*, 1992. **89**(13): 5951–55.

37. Logothetis, N. K. What we can do and what we cannot do with fMRI. *Nature*, 2008. **453**(7197): 869–78.

38. Logothetis, N. K. and Pfeuffer, J. On the nature of the BOLD fMRI contrast mechanism. *Magn Reson Imaging*, 2004. **22** (10): 1517–31.

39. Matthews, P. M., G. Honey, and E. Bullmore, Applications of fMRI in translational medicine and clinical practice. *Nat Neurosci*, 2006. **7**(9): 732–44.

40. Barch, D. M., et al., Working memory and prefrontal cortex dysfunction: specificity to schizophrenia compared with major depression. *Biol Psychiatry*, 2003. **53**(5): 376–84.

41. Greicius, M. D., et al., Resting-state functional connectivity in major depression: abnormally increased contributions from subgenual cingulate cortex and thalamus. *Biol Psychiatry*, 2007. **62**(5): 429–37.

42. Lagopoulos, J. and G. S. Malhi, A functional magnetic resonance imaging study of emotional Stroop in euthymic bipolar disorder. *Neuroreport*, 2007. **18**(15): 1583–87.

43. Honey, G. and E. Bullmore, Human pharmacological MRI. *Trends Pharmacol Sci*, 2004. **25**(7): 366–74.

44. Rauch, A., et al., Pharmacological MRI combined with electrophysiology in non-human primates: effects of Lidocaine on primary visual cortex. *Neuroimage*, 2008. **40**(2): 590–600.

45. Anderson, I. M., et al., Assessing human 5-HT function in vivo with pharmacoMRI. *Neuropharmacology*, 2008. **55**(6): 1029–37.

46. Martin, C. and N. R. Sibson, Pharmacological MRI in animal models: a useful tool for 5-HT research? *Neuropharmacology*, 2008. **55**(6): 1038–47.

47. King, J. A., et al., Procedure for minimizing stress for fMRI studies in conscious rats. *J Neurosci Methods*, 2005. **148**(2): 154–60.

48. Gottesman, I. I. and T. D. Gould, The endophenotype concept in psychiatry: etymology and strategic intentions. *Am J Psychiatry*, 2003. **160**(4): 636–45.

49. Frank, R. and R. Hargreaves, Clinical biomarkers in drug discovery and development. *Nat Rev Drug Discov*, 2003. **2**(7): 566–80.

50. Katz, R., Biomarkers and surrogate markers: an FDA perspective. *NeuroRx*, 2004. **1**(2): 189–95.

51. Mukhtar, M., Evolution of biomarkers: drug discovery to personalized medicine. *Drug Discov Today*, 2005. **10**(18): 1216–18.

52. Pien, H. H., et al., Using imaging biomarkers to accelerate drug development and clinical trials. *Drug Discov Today*, 2005. **10**(4): 259–66.

53. Bakhtiar, R., Biomarkers in drug discovery and development. *J Pharmacol Toxicol Methods*, 2008. **57**(2): 85–91.

54. Day, M., et al., Cognitive endpoints as disease biomarkers: optimizing the congruency of preclinical models to the clinic. *Curr Opin Investig Drugs*, 2008. **9**(7): 696–706.

55. Chan, S. W., et al., Risk for depression is associated with neural biases in emotional categorisation. *Neuropsychologia*, 2008. **46**(12): 2896–903.

56. Drevets, W. C., J. L. Price, and M. L. Furey, Brain structural and functional abnormalities in mood disorders: implications for neurocircuitry models of depression. *Brain Struct Func*, 2008. **213**(1–2):93–118.

57. Ekman, P. and W. V. Friesen, Constants across cultures in the face and emotion. *J Pers Soc Psychol*, 1971. **17**(2): 124–29.

58. Davidson, R. J., et al., The neural substrates of affective processing in depressed patients treated with venlafaxine. *Am J Psychiatry*, 2003. **160**(1): 64–75.

59. Davidson, R. J., et al., Depression: perspectives from affective neuroscience. *Annu Rev Psychol*, 2002. **53**: 545–74.

60. Hamilton, J. P. and I. H. Gotlib, Neural substrates of increased memory sensitivity for negative stimuli in major depression. *Biol Psychiatry*, 2008. **63**(12): 1155–62.

61. Anand, A., et al. Antidepressant effect on connectivity of the mood-regulating circuit: an FMRI study. *Neuropsychopharmacology*, 2005. **30**(7): 1334–44.

62. Johnstone, T., et al., Stability of amygdala BOLD response to fearful faces over multiple scan sessions. *NeuroImage*, 2005. **25**(4): 1112–23.

63. Fu, C. H., et al., Attenuation of the neural response to sad faces in major depression by antidepressant treatment: a prospective, event-related functional magnetic resonance imaging study. *Arch Gen Psychiatry*, 2004. **61**(9): 877–89.

64. Joormann, J. and M. Siemer, Memory accessibility, mood regulation, and dysphoria: difficulties in repairing sad mood with happy memories? *J Abnorm Psychol*, 2004. **113**(2): 179–88.

65. Gilboa-Schechtman, E., D. Erhard-Weiss, and P. Jeczemien, Interpersonal deficits meet cognitive biases: memory for facial expressions in depressed and anxious men and women. *Psychiatry Res*, 2002. **113**(3): 279–93.

66. Anand, A., et al., Activity and connectivity of brain mood regulating circuit in depression: a functional magnetic resonance study. *Biol Psychiatry*, 2005. **57**(10): 1079–88.

67. Berg, E. A., A simple objective technique for measuring flexibility in thinking. *J Gen Psychol*, 1948. **39**: 15–22.

68. Kirchner, W. K., Age differences in short-term retention of rapidly changing information. *J Exp Psychol*, 1958. **55**(4): 352–58.

69. Kiloh, L. G., Pseudo-dementia. *Acta Psychiatr Scand*, 1961. **37**: 336–51.

70. Zakzanis, K. K., L. Leach, and E. Kaplan, On the nature and pattern of neurocognitive function in major depressive disorder. *Neuropsychiatry Neuropsychol Behav Neurol*, 1998. **11**(3): 111–19.

71. van Gorp, W. G., et al., Cognitive impairment in euthymic bipolar patients with and without prior alcohol dependence. A preliminary study. *Arch Gen Psychiatry*, 1998. **55**(1): 41–46.

72. Veiel, H. O., A preliminary profile of neuropsychological deficits associated with major depression. *J Clin Exp Neuropsychol*, 1997. **19**(4): 587–603.

73. Paterniti, S., et al., Anxiety, depression, psychotropic drug use and cognitive impairment. *Psychol Med*, 1999. **29**(2): 421–28.

74. Wadsworth, E. J., et al., SSRIs and cognitive performance in a working sample. *Hum Psychopharmacol*, 2005. **20**(8): 561–72.

75. Harlow, H. and J. Bromer, A test apparatus for monkeys. *Psychol Rec*, 1939. **2**: 434–36.

76. Hoffman, K. L., et al., Facial-expression and gaze-selective responses in the monkey amygdala. *Curr Biol*, 2007. **17**(9): 766–72.

77. Passingham, R., How good is the macaque monkey model of the human brain? *Curr Opin Neurobiol*, 2009. **19**(1): 6–11.

78. Preuss, T. M., Do rats have prefrontal cortex? The Rose–Woolsey–Akert program reconsidered. *J Cogn Neurosci*, 1995. **7**(1): 1–24.

79. Campbell, M., et al., RNAi-mediated reversible opening of the blood–brain barrier. *J Gene Med*, 2008. **10**(8): 930–47.

80. Cho, Z. H., et al., A fusion PET-MRI system with a high-resolution research tomograph-PET and ultra-high field 7.0 T-MRI for the molecular-genetic imaging of the brain. *Proteomics*, 2008. **8**(6): 1302–23.

81. Ruhé, H. G., et al., Serotonin transporter gene promoter polymorphisms modify the association between paroxetine serotonin transporter occupancy and clinical response in major depressive disorder. *Pharmacogenet Genomics*, 2009. **19**(1): 67–76.

82. Smith, D. F. and S. Jakobsen, Molecular tools for assessing human depression by positron emission tomography. *Eur Neuropsychopharmacol*, 2009. **19**(9): 611–28.

83. Ross, J. S., et al., Pharmacogenomics and clinical biomarkers in drug discovery and development. *Am J Clin Pathol*, 2005. **124** Suppl: S29–41.

84. Kato, T., Molecular genetics of bipolar disorder and depression. *Psychiatry Clin Neurosci*, 2007. **61**(1): 3–19.

85. Maier, W., Common risk genes for affective and schizophrenic psychoses. *Eur Arch Psychiatry Clin Neurosci*, 2008. **258**(S2): 37–40.

86. Caspi, A., et al., Influence of life stress on depression: moderation by a polymorphism in the 5-HTT gene. *Science*, 2003. **301**(5631): 386–89.

87. Hayden, E. P., et al., Early emerging cognitive vulnerability to depression and the serotonin transporter promoter region polymorphism. *J Affect Disord*, 2008. **107**(1–3): 227–30.

88. Collier, D., et al., A novel functional polymorphism within the promoter of the serotonin transporter gene: possible role in susceptibility to affective disorders. *Mol Psychiatry*, 1996. **1**(6): 453–60.

89. Willis-Owen, S. A., et al., The serotonin transporter length polymorphism, neuroticism, and depression: a comprehensive assessment of association. *Biol Psychiatry*, 2005. **58**(6): 451–56.

90. Wilson, M. E. and B. Kinkead, Gene–environment interactions, not neonatal growth hormone deficiency, time puberty in female rhesus monkeys. *Biol Reprod*, 2008. **78**(4): 736–43.

91. Jarrell, H., et al., Polymorphisms in the serotonin reuptake transporter gene modify the consequences of social status on metabolic health in female rhesus monkeys. *Physiol Behav*, 2008. **93**(4–5): 807–19.

92. Bethea, C. L., et al., Anxious behavior and fenfluramine-induced prolactin secretion in young rhesus macaques with different alleles of the serotonin reuptake transporter polymorphism (5HTTLPR). *Behav Genet*, 2004. **34**(3): 295–307.

93. Hariri, A. R., et al., Serotonin transporter genetic variation and the response of the human amygdala. *Science*, 2002. **297**(5580): 400–03.

94. Hariri, A. R., et al., A susceptibility gene for affective disorders and the response of the human amygdala. *Arch Gen Psychiatry*, 2005. **62**(2): 146–52.

95. Pezawas, L., et al., 5-HTTLPR polymorphism impacts human cingulate-amygdala interactions: a genetic susceptibility mechanism for depression. *Nat Neurosci*, 2005. **8**(6): 828–34.

96. David, S. P., et al., A functional genetic variation of the serotonin (5-HT) transporter affects 5-HT1A receptor binding in humans. *J Neurosci*, 2005. **25**(10): 2586–90.

97. Willeit, M., et al. No evidence for in vivo regulations of midbrain serotonin transporter availability by serotonin transporter promoter gene polymorphism. *Biol Psychiatry*, 2001. **50**(1): 8–12.

98. Shioe, K., et al. No association between genotype of the promoter region of serotonin transporter gene and serotonin transporter binding in human brain measured by PET. *Synapse*, 2003. **48**(4): 184–88.

99. Pezawas, L., et al., Evidence of biologic epistasis between BDNF and SLC6A4 and implications for depression. *Mol Psychiatry*, 2008. **13**(7): 709–16.

100. Frank, R. and R. Hargreaves, Clinical biomarkers in drug discovery and development. *Nat Rev Drug Discov*, 2003. **2**(7): 566–80.

101. Meyerlindenberg, A., et al., False positives in imaging genetics. *Neuroimage*, 2008. **8**(2): 655–61.

102. Gardier, A. M., Mutant mouse models and antidepressant drug research: focus on serotonin and brain-derived neurotrophic factor. *Behav Pharmacol*, 2009. **20**(1): 18–32.

103. Kato, T., et al., Behavioral and gene expression analyses of Wfs1 knockout mice as a possible animal model of mood disorder. *Neurosci Res*, 2008. **61**(2): 143–58.

104. Bearer, E. L., et al., Reward circuitry is perturbed in the absence of the serotonin transporter. *NeuroImage*, 2009. **46**(4): 1091–104.

105. Willmann, J. K., et al., Molecular imaging in drug development. *Nat Rev Drug Discov*, 2008. **7**(7): 591–607.

106. Hume, S. P., R. N. Gunn, and T. Jones, Pharmacological constraints associated with positron emission tomographic scanning of small laboratory animals. *Eur J Nucl Med*, 1998. **25**(2): 173–76.

107. Sossi, V. and T. J. Ruth, Micropet imaging: in vivo biochemistry in small animals. *J Neural Transm*, 2005. **112**(3): 319–30.

108. Pardridge, W. M., The blood–brain barrier: bottleneck in brain drug development. *NeuroRx*, 2005. **2**(1): 3–14.

109. Pardridge, W. M., Blood–brain barrier drug targeting: the future of brain drug development. *Mol Interv*, 2003. **3**(2): 90–105, 51.

110. Meyer, J. H., Imaging the serotonin transporter during major depressive disorder and antidepressant treatment. *J Psychiatry Neurosci*, 2007. **32**(2) 86–102.

111. Andrée, B., et al., Use of PET and the radioligand [carbonyl-(11)C]WAY-100635 in psychotropic drug development. *Nucl Med Biol*, 2000. **27**(5): 515–21.

112. Lemaire, C., et al., Fluorine-18-altanserin: a radioligand for the study of serotonin receptors with PET: radiolabeling and in vivo biologic behavior in rats. *J Nucl Med*, 1991. **32**(12): 2266–72.

113. Kato, T., T. Inubushi, and N. Kato, Magnetic resonance spectroscopy in

affective disorders. *J Neuropsychiatry Clin Neurosci*, 1998. **10**(2): 133–47.

114. Bolo, N. R., et al., Brain pharmacokinetics and tissue distribution in vivo of fluvoxamine and fluoxetine by fluorine magnetic resonance spectroscopy. *Neuropsychopharmacology*, 2000. **23**(4): 428–38.

115. Henry, M. E., et al., A comparison of brain and serum pharmacokinetics of *R*-fluoxetine and racemic fluoxetine: a 19-F MRS study. *Neuropsychopharmacology*, 2005. **30**(8): 1576–83.

116. Chen, C. H., et al., Brain imaging correlates of depressive symptom severity and predictors of symptom improvement after antidepressant treatment. *Biol Psychiatry*, 2007. **62**(5): 407–14.

117. Frankel, R. J., J. S. Jenkins, and J. J. Wright, Pituitary–adrenal response to stimulation of the limbic system and lateral hypothalamus in the rhesus monkey (*Macacca mulatta*). *Acta Endocrinol*, 1978. **88**(2): 209–16.

118. Kalin, N. H., S. Shelton, and R. J. Davidson, The role of the central nucleus of the amygdala in mediating fear and anxiety in the primate. *J Neurosci*, 2004. **24**(24): 5506–15.

119. Machado, C. J. and J. Bachevalier, Behavioral and hormonal reactivity to threat: effects of selective amygdala, hippocampal or orbital frontal lesions in monkeys. *Psychoneuroendocrinology*, 2008. **33**(7): 926–41.

120. Sapolsky, R. M., L. C. Krey, and B. S. McEwen, Glucocorticoid-sensitive hippocampal neurons are involved in terminating the adrenocortical stress response. *Proc Natl Acad Sci USA*, 1984. **81**(19): 6174–77.

121. Feldman, S. and J. Weidenfeld, Electrical stimulation of the dorsal hippocampus caused a long lasting inhibition of ACTH and adrenocortical responses to photic stimuli in freely moving rats. *Brain Res*, 2001. **911**(1): 22–26.

122. Goursaud, A. P., S. P. Mendoza, and J. P. Capitanio, Do neonatal bilateral ibotenic acid lesions of the hippocampal

formation or of the amygdala impair HPA axis responsiveness and regulation in infant rhesus macaques (*Macaca mulatta*)? *Brain Res*, 2006. **1071**(1): 97–104.

123. Halbreich, U., et al., Cortisol secretion in endogenous depression. I. Basal plasma levels. *Arch Gen Psychiatry*, 1985. **42**(9): 904–08.

124. Stokes, P. E., et al., Pretreatment DST and hypothalamic–pituitary–adrenocortical function in depressed patients and comparison groups. A multicenter study. *Arch Gen Psychiatry*, 1984. **41**(3): 257–67.

125. Heuser, I., A. Yassouridis, and F. Holsboer, The combined dexamethasone/CRH test: a refined laboratory test for psychiatric disorders. *J Psychiatr Res*, 1994. **28**(4): 341–56.

126. Holsboer, F., et al., Stimulation response to corticotropin-releasing hormone (CRH) in patients with depression, alcoholism and panic disorder. *Horm Metab Res Suppl*, 1987. **16**: 80–88.

127. Kitamura, Y., H. Araki, and Y. Gomita, Influence of ACTH on the effects of imipramine, desipramine and lithium on duration of immobility of rats in the forced swim test. *Pharmacol Biochem Behav*, 2002. **71**(1–2): 63–69.

128. Kitamura, Y., et al., Effects of imipramine and bupropion on the duration of immobility of ACTH-treated rats in the forced swim test: involvement of the expression of 5-HT2A receptor mRNA. *Biol Pharm Bull*, 2008. **31**(2): 246–49.

129. Kaufman, I. C. and L. A. Rosenblum, Depression in infant monkeys separated from their mothers. *Science*, 1967. **155**(765): 1030–31.

130. Kaufman, I. C. and L. A. Rosenblum, The reaction to separation in infant monkeys: anaclitic depression and conservation-withdrawal. *Psychosom Med*, 1967. **29**(6): 648–75.

131. Harlow, H. F., P. E. Plubell, and C. M. Baysinger, Induction of psychological death in rhesus monkeys. *J Autism Child Schizophr*, 1973. **3**(4): 299–307.

132. Young, L. D., et al., Early stress and later response to separation in rhesus monkeys. *Am J Psychiatry*, 1973. **130**(4): 400–05.

133. Harlow, H. F. and S. J. Suomi, Induced depression in monkeys. *Behav Biol*, 1974. **12**(3): 273–96.

134. Suomi, S. J., et al., Depressive behavior in adult monkeys following separation from family environment. *J Abnorm Psychol*, 1975. **84**(5): 576–78.

135. Kalin, N. H., et al., Brain regions associated with the expression and contextual regulation of anxiety in primates. *Biol Psychiatry*, 2005. **58**(10): 796–804.

136. Bennett, A. J., et al., Early experience and serotonin transporter gene variation interact to influence primate CNS function. *Mol Psychiatry*, 2002. **7**(1): 118–22.

137. Suomi, S. J., Risk, resilience, and gene × environment interactions in rhesus monkeys. *Ann NY Acad Sci*, 2006. **1094**: 52–62.

138. Kalin, N. H., et al., The serotonin transporter genotype is associated with intermediate brain phenotypes that depend on the context of eliciting stressor. *Mol Psychiatry*, 2008. **13**(11): 1021–27.

139. Mackay, T. F. and R. R. Anholt, Ain't misbehavin' ? Genotype-environment interactions and the genetics of behavior. *Trends Genet*, 2007. **23**(7): 311–14.

140. Gotlib, I. H., et al., HPA axis reactivity: a mechanism underlying the associations among 5-HTTLPR, stress, and depression. *Biol Psychiatry*, 2008. **63**(9): 847–51.

141. Malberg, J. E. and J. A. Blendy, Antidepressant action: to the nucleus and beyond. *Trends Pharmacol Sci*, 2005. **26**(12): 631–38.

142. Krishnan, V. and E. Nestler, The molecular neurobiology of depression. *Nature*, 2008. **455**(7215): 894–902.

143. Roffman, J. L., et al., Neuroimaging-genetic paradigms: a new approach to investigate the pathophysiology and treatment of cognitive deficits in schizophrenia. *Harvard Rev Psychiatry*, 2006. **14**(2): 78–91.

144. Savitz, J. B. and W. C. Drevets, Imaging phenotypes of major depressive disorder: genetic correlates. *Neuroscience*, 2009. **164**(1): 300–30.

145. Sklar, P., et al., Family based association study of 76 candidate genes in bipolar disorder: BDNF is a potential risk locus. Brain-derived neutrophic factor. *Mol Psychiatry*, 2002. **7**(6): 579–93.

146. Neves-Pereira, M., et al., The brain-derived neurotrophic factor gene confers susceptibility to bipolar disorder: evidence from a family based association study. *Am J Hum Genet*, 2002. **71**(3): 651–55.

147. Green, E. K., et al., Genetic variation of brain-derived neurotrophic factor (BDNF) in bipolar disorder: case-control study of over 3000 individuals from the UK. *Br J Psychiatry*, 2006. **188**: 21–25.

148. Hariri, A. R., et al., Brain-derived neurotrophic factor val66met polymorphism affects human memory-related hippocampal activity and predicts memory performance. *J Neurosci*, 2003. **23**(17): 6690–94.

149. Egan, M. F., et al., The BDNF val66met polymorphism affects activity-dependent secretion of BDNF and human memory and hippocampal function. *Cell*, 2003. **112**(2): 257–69.

150. Frey, B. N., et al., Brain-derived neurotrophic factor val66met polymorphism affects prefrontal energy metabolism in bipolar disorder. *Neuroreport*, 2007. **18**(15): 1567–70.

151. Rybakowski, J. K., et al., Polymorphism of the brain-derived neurotrophic factor gene and performance on a cognitive prefrontal test in bipolar patients. *Bipolar Disord*, 2003. **5**(6): 468–72.

152. Fukumoto, T., et al., Chronic lithium treatment increases the expression of brain-derived neurotrophic factor in the rat brain. *Psychopharmacology*, 2001. **158**(1): 100–06.

153. Alme, M. N., et al., Chronic fluoxetine treatment induces brain region-specific upregulation of genes associated with BDNF-induced long-term potentiation. *Neural Plast*, 2007. **2007**: 26496.

154. Gratacòs, M., et al., Brain-derived neurotrophic factor Val66Met and psychiatric disorders: meta-analysis of

case-control studies confirm association to substance-related disorders, eating disorders, and schizophrenia. *Biol Psychiatry*, 2007. **61**(7): 911–22.

155. Rybakowski, J. K., et al., Prophylactic lithium response and polymorphism of the brain-derived neurotrophic factor gene. *Pharmacopsychiatry*, 2005. **38**(4): 166–70.

156. Yoshida, K., et al., The G196A polymorphism of the brain-derived neurotrophic factor gene and the antidepressant effect of milnacipran and fluvoxamine. *J Psychopharmacol (Oxford)*, 2007. **21**(6): 650–56.

157. Tsai, S. J., et al., Association study of a brain-derived neurotrophic-factor genetic polymorphism and major depressive disorders, symptomatology, and antidepressant response. *Am J Med Genet B Neuropsychiatr Genet*, 2003. **123B**(1): 19–22.

158. Choi, M. J., et al., Brain-derived neurotrophic factor gene polymorphism (Val66Met) and citalopram response in major depressive disorder. *Brain Res*, 2006. **1118**(1): 176–82.

159. Rybakowski, J. K., et al., Response to lithium prophylaxis: interaction between serotonin transporter and BDNF genes. *Am J Med Genet B Neuropsychiatr Genet*, 2007. **144B**(6): 820–23.

160. Capuron, L. and R. Dantzer, Cytokines and depression: the need for a new paradigm. *Brain Behav Immun*, 2003. **17** Suppl 1: S119–24.

161. Miller, A. H., V. Maletic, and C. L. Raison, Inflammation and its discontents: the role of cytokines in the pathophysiology of major depression. *Biol Psychiatry*, 2009. **65**(9): 732–41.

162. Hickie, I. and A. Lloyd, Are cytokines associated with neuropsychiatric syndromes in humans? *Int J Immunopharmacol*, 1995. **17**(8): 677–83.

163. Hickie, I., et al., Biochemical correlates of in vivo cell-mediated immune dysfunction in patients with depression: a preliminary report. *Int J Immunopharmacol*, 1995. **17**(8): 685–90.

164. Capuron, L., et al., Treatment of cytokine-induced depression. *Brain Behav Immun*, 2002. **16**(5): 575–80.

165. Felger, J. C., et al., Effects of interferon-alpha on rhesus monkeys: a nonhuman primate model of cytokine-induced depression. *Biol Psychiatry*, 2007. **62**(11): 1324–33.

166. Larson, S. J., et al., Effects of interleukin-1beta on food-maintained behavior in the mouse. *Brain Behav Immun*, 2002. **16**(4): 398–410.

167. Mendlewicz, J., et al., Shortened onset of action of antidepressants in major depression using acetylsalicylic acid augmentation: a pilot open-label study. *Int Clin Psychopharmacol*, 2006. **21**(4): 227–31.

168. Muller, N., et al., The cyclooxygenase-2 inhibitor celecoxib has therapeutic effects in major depression: results of a double-blind, randomized, placebo controlled, add-on pilot study to reboxetine. *Mol Psychiatry*, 2006. **11**(7): 680–84.

169. Harrison, N. A., et al., Neural origins of human sickness in interoceptive responses to inflammation. *Biol Psychiatry*, 2009. **66**(5): 415–22.

170. Harrison, N. A., et al., Inflammation causes mood changes through alterations in subgenual cingulate activity, and mesolimbic connectivity. *Biol Psychiatry*, 2009. **66**(5): 407–14.

171. Brydon, L., et al., Peripheral inflammation is associated with altered substantia nigra activity and psychomotor slowing in humans. *Biol Psychiatry*, 2008. **63**(11): 1022–29.

172. Mayberg, H. S., et al., Reciprocal limbic–cortical function and negative mood: converging PET findings in depression and normal sadness. *Am J Psychiatry*, 1999. **156**(5): 675–82.

173. Alexopoulos, G. S., et al., 'Vascular depression' hypothesis. *Arch Gen Psychiatry*, 1997. **54**(10): 915–22.

174. Steffens, D. C. and K. R. Krishnan, Structural neuroimaging and mood disorders: recent findings, implications for classification, and future directions. *Biol Psychiatry*, 1998. **43**(10): 705–12.

175. Alexopoulos, G. S., Frontostriatal and limbic dysfunction in late-life depression. *Am J Geriatr Psychiatry*, 2002. **10**(6): 687–95.

176. Alexopoulos, G. S., et al., Clinical presentation of the "depression–executive dysfunction syndrome" of late life. *Am J Geriatr Psychiatry*, 2002. **10**(1): 98–106.

177. Alexopoulos, G. S., The vascular depression hypothesis: 10 years later. *Biol Psychiatry*, 2006. **60**(12): 1304–05.

178. Simpson, S., et al., Is subcortical disease associated with a poor response to antidepressants? Neurological, neuropsychological and neuroradiological findings in late-life depression. *Psychol Med*, 1998. **28**(5): 1015–26.

179. Hickie, I., et al., Subcortical hyperintensities on magnetic resonance imaging: clinical correlates and prognostic significance in patients with severe depression. *Biol Psychiatry*, 1995. **37**(3): 151–60.

180. Simpson, S., et al., Subcortical vascular disease in elderly patients with treatment resistant depression. *J Neurol, Neurosurg Psychiatry*, 1997. **62**(2): 196–97.

181. Potter, G. G., et al., Prefrontal neuropsychological predictors of treatment remission in late-life depression. *Neuropsychopharmacology*, 2004. **29**(12): 2266–71.

182. Ernst, E., Placebo: new insights into an old enigma. *Drug Discov Today*, 2007. **12**(9–10): 413–18.

183. Walsh, B. T., et al., Placebo response in studies of major depression: variable, substantial, and growing. *JAMA*, 2002. **287**(14): 1840–47.

184. Kirsch, I., Challenging received wisdom: antidepressants and the placebo effect. *Mcgill J Med*, 2008. **11**(2): 219–22.

185. Brunoni, A. R., et al., Placebo response of non-pharmacological and pharmacological trials in major depression: a systematic review and meta-analysis. *PLoS ONE*, 2009. **4**(3): e4824.

186. Lidstone, S. C. and A. J. Stoessl, Understanding the placebo effect: contributions from neuroimaging. *Molec Imaging Biol*, 2007. **9**(4): 176–85.

187. Mayberg, H. S., et al., The functional neuroanatomy of the placebo effect. *Am J Psychiatry*, 2002. **159**(5): 728–37.

188. Mayberg, H. S., et al., Regional metabolic effects of fluoxetine in major depression: serial changes and relationship to clinical response. *Biol Psychiatry*, 2000. **48**(8): 830–43.

189. Leuchter, A. F., et al., Changes in brain function of depressed subjects during treatment with placebo. *Am J Psychiatry*, 2002. **159**(1): 122–29.

Chapter 5

Defining depression endophenotypes

Lisa H. Berghorst and Diego A. Pizzagalli

Abstract

It is widely assumed that major depressive disorder (MDD) includes a heterogeneous mix of conditions reached through multiple etiological and pathophysiological processes. In recent years, efforts to parse the heterogeneity inherent to MDD have led to renewed interest in identifying potential depressive "endophenotypes" – intermediate phenotypes hypothesized to lie within the etiological link between genes and clinical disease. In this chapter, we begin with an overview of the endophenotype concept and its central criteria (clinical and biological plausibility, specificity, state-independence, heritability, familial association, and cosegregation). Next, we examine the potential utility of applying an endophenotypic approach to depression research, with a focus on anhedonia as a particularly promising depressive endophenotype. To this end, we review and integrate findings across epidemiological, behavioral, neuroimaging, and genetic studies to assess anhedonia within the endophenotypic criteria. Following this examination, we discuss current directions in the development of objective laboratory-based measures of anhedonia and their value in facilitating a more precise identification of the psychological and neurobiological mechanisms underlying anhedonia. We conclude that utilizing an endophenotypic approach may improve our understanding of the etiology and pathophysiology of depression, which would ultimately enhance our ability to design more effective treatment and prevention strategies.

Introduction

Major depressive disorder (MDD) is a highly prevalent and recurrent illness that is a leading cause of disease burden across the world [1]. In the United States alone, for example, the lifetime prevalence rate has been estimated to be 16.6%, affecting over 30 million people, with more than 80% of these individuals experiencing recurrent episodes [2,3]. At both the individual and population levels, depression engenders severe impairment in functioning across social, cognitive, and occupational domains [4,5]. Given the pervasive and detrimental effects of depression, it is disconcerting that in the largest prospective treatment study to date (the Sequenced Treatment Alternatives to Relieve Depression (STAR*D) study), only about one-third of participants remitted after treatment with a standard, first-line antidepressant (the selective serotonin reuptake inhibitor (SSRI) citalopram), and the probability of remission generally decreased over subsequent treatment levels [6]. Unfortunately, efforts to design more effective treatment strategies for depression are limited by the fact that the etiological pathways underlying this disorder remain complex and elusive.

Next Generation Antidepressants: Moving Beyond Monoamines to Discover Novel Treatment Strategies for Mood Disorders, ed. Chad E. Beyer and Stephen M. Stahl. Published by Cambridge University Press.
© Cambridge University Press 2010.

In recent years, concerns have been raised that the ongoing quest to understand the etiology and pathophysiology of MDD might be hindered in part by difficulties in defining and characterizing psychiatric phenotypes (e.g. [7–9]). With respect to MDD, it has been suggested that the current classification criteria encompass a heterogeneous mix of illnesses that share similar final pathways likely reached via multiple pathophysiological processes [7]. One way to address this heterogeneity is to take an "endophenotypic" approach and focus on intermediate phenotypes that are more narrowly defined and quantified than DSM-IV diagnoses [10].

Our goal in this chapter is to summarize literature on the potential utility of applying an endophenotypic approach to depression research, with a focus on one of the most promising depressive endophenotypes – anhedonia, defined as loss of pleasure or lack of reactivity to pleasurable stimuli [11]. We begin with an overview of the endophenotype concept and its central criteria, which include the following [7,10]: (1) biological and clinical plausibility, (2) specificity, (3) state-independence, (4) familial association, (5) cosegregation, and (6) heritability. In depression research, various endophenotypes have been proposed and assessed with respect to these criteria, including impaired reward function (anhedonia), impaired learning and memory, increased stress sensitivity, REM sleep abnormalities, and tryptophan depletion, among others (see [7] for review). Our focus in this chapter will be on anhedonia, as it has received some of the strongest empirical evidence [7,12,13]. To this end, we incorporate epidemiological, behavioral, neuroimaging, and genetic studies to examine the aforementioned endophenotypic criteria for anhedonia. Thereafter, we discuss an objective way to measure anhedonia in a laboratory setting and summarize recent findings using this paradigm. The chapter concludes with a discussion of important directions for future research efforts using an endophenotypic approach.

The endophenotype concept in relation to psychiatry

Definition and value of endophenotypes

The identification of etiological and pathophysiological processes underlying mental disorders has proven to be an exceptionally difficult mission, and these processes remain largely unknown despite vigorous research efforts over several decades. As previously noted, a substantial contributing factor to this difficulty may be the structure of current classification systems, including the *Diagnostic and Statistical Manual of Mental Disorders* (DSM-IV; [11]), in which the diagnosis of mental disorders revolves around symptom clusters and clinical course [7,9]. This descriptive, categorical approach is implemented in an effort to maximize diagnostic reliability; however, it brings the issue of validity into question for various mental disorders, including MDD [14]. As a result of the organizational framework of the DSM-IV, these categories of disorders may encompass a heterogeneous mix of illnesses [7,15]. The heterogeneity of clinical phenotypes is postulated to reflect the involvement of a multitude of genes – none of which is likely necessary or sufficient for triggering a given disorder – as well as complex interactions between genes and environmental factors [10,16,17]. In response to this issue of heterogeneity, one approach is to focus research efforts on "endophenotypes," or intermediate phenotypes that are hypothesized to lie within the etiological link between genes and clinical disease [8,10]. Accordingly, the endophenotypic approach enables the identification of "the 'upstream' consequences of genes" as well as "the 'downstream' traits or facets of clinical phenotypes" [p. 637; 10]. One assumption underlying this conceptualization is that endophenotypes involve comparatively fewer genes and enable a more direct measurement of the biological and environmental factors that contribute to a disorder than afforded by the broader perspective of the clinical phenotype [10]. This assumption was recently challenged by Flint and Mufano [18], who contended that some endophenotypes may not be considerably less genetically complex than clinical disease phenotypes, raising potential concerns about the "incremental" validity of the endophenotypic approach with respect to genetic architecture. While this concern is legitimate, it is important to recognize that the conclusions drawn by Flint and Mufano were predominantly based on results restricted to the effects of Catechd-*O*-methyltransferense (COMT) genotype on endopheno-types, which may limit the generalizability of their conclusion. Moreover, Flint and Mufano acknowledge that an endophenotypic approach may still be beneficial to genetic research and contribute to higher reliability across data by enabling objective quantitative measures to be obtained from the large number of individuals necessary for genetic analyses. Nevertheless, additional research is clearly needed to evaluate the incremental validity of the endopheno-typic approach, particularly with respect to etiological pathways underlying mental illnesses. Ultimately, these endeavors could have vast implications for improving the validity of our classification system and the effectiveness of treatment and prevention methods.

Criteria and validation of endophenotypes

Putative endophenotypes can be examined using psychological, physiological, neuroimag-ing, and biochemical methods [7]. In order for a psychological or biological variable to be classified as an endophenotype, it should meet the following criteria [7,10,19,20]:

1. *Clinical and biological plausibility*: Conceptual relationships exist between the endophenotype and the disease of interest.

2. *Specificity*: The endophenotype is linked more strongly to the psychiatric disorder of interest than to other psychiatric disorders.[1]

3. *State-independence*: The endophenotype is stable over time and not dependent on illness status or treatment. In other words, the endophenotype should be apparent in an individual regardless of whether or not (s)he is actively experiencing symptoms of the illness.[2]

4. *Heritability*: A proportion of variance in the endophenotype is attributable to genetic variance.

5. *Familial association*: The endophenotype occurs more frequently in unaffected relatives of ill individuals than in the general population.

6. *Cosegregation*: Within families of ill individuals, the endophenotype occurs more frequently in family members who are affected with the illness than in family members who are unaffected by the illness.

In addition to the aforementioned criteria, it is important to take into account the degree to which a putative endophenotype can be feasibly and reliably measured [15]. Along these lines, in the section "*Current directions in objective laboratory measurements of anhedonia*,"

---

[1] Hasler and colleagues [15] recently suggested that the specificity criterion might not be necessary because the biological validity of current definitions of mental disorders remains under question.

[2] In an attempt to take into account developmental factors and symptom provocation methods in phenotypic expression, Hasler and colleagues [15] subsequently modified this criterion to state that it may be age-normed and may require an environmental challenge to be apparent.

we will describe our experience utilizing a laboratory-based measure to objectively assess an important component of anhedonia (reward responsiveness).

Anhedonia as a potential depressive endophenotype

The notion that anhedonia may be a trait marker of vulnerability to depression has been under consideration for many years [21–23]. Within the past decade in particular, anhedonia has received considerable support as a promising depressive endophenotype [7,12,13]. As summarized in the following sections, empirical evidence supports the endophenotypic criteria of clinical and biological plausibility, familial association, and heritability; mixed or limited findings exist for state-independence and specificity, and few studies have addressed cosegregation. Throughout these sections, the emphasis will be on studies that include laboratory-based tasks in addition to self-report measures, rather than studies focusing exclusively on the latter.

Clinical and biological plausibility of anhedonia as a depressive endophenotype

Among the DSM-IV criteria for a major depressive episode, anhedonia is a cardinal symptom with comparable status as depressed mood, given that one of these two features is required for clinical diagnosis [11]. In order to more explicitly understand the role of anhedonia in depression, researchers have examined a variety of domains, including affective and behavioral responses to positive stimuli, perceptual and attentional processing of positive cues, and ability to learn from reinforcement history. Investigations have also been conducted to examine whether anhedonic symptoms have predictive validity with regard to clinical outcome. Moreover, neuroimaging studies have been utilized to explore relationships between abnormal functioning within particular reward-related brain regions and depression. In the ensuing sections, findings stemming from these lines of inquiry will be considered in order to evaluate the clinical and biological plausibility of anhedonia as a depressive endophenotype.

In an early study probing the encoding of positive stimuli, Berenbaum and Oltmanns [24] found that depressed individuals, relative to healthy controls, reported less positive affect and displayed fewer positive facial expressions when presented with positive film clips. Along similar lines, Sloan and colleagues [25] reported that depressed participants rated pleasant picture stimuli less positively, and displayed reduced frequency and intensity of pleasant facial expressions, compared to controls. Importantly, in both studies, findings were selective to positive stimuli and did not extend to negative stimuli. Evidence of reduced facial reactivity (e.g. [26,27]) and affective responses (e.g. [28–31]) to positive stimuli has emerged from additional studies, although null findings have also been described (e.g. [32,33]). If present, blunted affective and behavioral reactivity to positive stimuli could arguably influence subsequent retrieval of such stimuli. However, before discussing studies on retrieval, it is worth considering perceptual and attentional processing of positive cues, as these processes could arguably also influence retrieval.

In the realm of perceptual processing, findings are inconsistent regarding whether depressed individuals are impaired in their ability to recognize positive stimuli, such as happy facial expressions. Various researchers report no impairment on face recognition tasks in depression (e.g. [34–36]). Meanwhile, others have found that depressed individuals, relative to controls, are less accurate in recognizing happy facial expressions (e.g. [37,38]), and require more time (e.g. [39]) and greater intensity of emotional expression (e.g. [40]) in order to label faces as happy. Of note, recognition impairment was specific to positive facial stimuli only in the latter two studies [39,40]. Discrepancies across the aforementioned results may be due in part to the heterogeneous nature of depression, or to the possibility that some results may be confounded by response biases, especially if only accuracy and reaction time were measured.

There is also mixed evidence with respect to attentional biases in depression. In several studies using the deployment-of-attention (e.g. [41,42]) or dot-probe [43] paradigms, depressed patients failed to show the positivity bias seen in healthy controls, who directed their attention toward positive stimuli. While these studies lend credence towards a depression-related attentional bias away from positive stimuli, others report null findings (e.g. [44]). Nevertheless, a potentially blunted attentional positivity bias, along with possible impairments in recognizing positive stimuli, and reduced affective and behavioral reactivity to positive stimuli at encoding, may all impede the ability of depressed individuals to retrieve positive cues. Indeed, depressed individuals are more likely to underestimate the occurrence of positive reinforcements received in the past (e.g. [45,46]). It is important to note that this pattern of impairment does not extend to estimations of punishments, as depressed individuals are actually more likely to overestimate the occurrence of punishments received in the past [46]. Furthermore, a biased view of past positive experiences may contribute towards a biased calculation of future outcomes, since individuals with depression also report lower expectations of positive future experiences than control subjects (e.g. [47,48]).

Findings of underestimation of past positive reinforcements received may be related to emerging data in which depressed subjects display a reduced ability to modify behavior as a function of positive reinforcements received, as evident from a monetarily reinforced verbal recognition task [49,50], a gambling task [51], and a probabilistic reward task [13; see section on: *Current directions in objective laboratory measurements of anhedonia*]. In sum, the above studies provide evidence that depression is characterized by: reduced affective and behavioral reactivity to positive stimuli; underestimation of the occurrence of past, and the likelihood of future, positive reinforcements; and a reduced ability to use reinforcement history to modify behavior. Evidence of blunted perceptual and attentional processing biases is more tenuous (see also [52]).

Of clinical relevance, anhedonic symptoms and behaviors have been found to have predictive value in determining depression onset, course, and outcome, as discussed hereafter. For example, reduced frequency of choosing high-magnitude reward options in a decision-making task predicted depressive symptoms one year later in a pediatric sample [51]. With respect to predicting levels of concurrent depressive symptoms, lower levels of approach-related behavior – but not higher levels of avoidance-related behavior – have been associated with increased severity of depression in currently depressed individuals [53]. Along these lines, lower levels of approach-related behavior [53,54], lower behavioral and heart rate reactivity to amusing films [55], and reduced recall of positive words [56] have been found to predict poorer longitudinal outcome and/or longer time to recovery in depressed individuals. Complementing such studies, Lethbridge and Allen [57] conducted a prospective study in a community sample of individuals with past depression and reported that larger levels of reduced positive affect following a sad mood induction correlated with a greater probability of MDD recurrence a year later; notably, relapse was not predicted by changes in negative affect or dysfunctional thinking, indicating specificity.

Finally, additional support for anhedonia as a potential vulnerability factor for the development of depression comes from the fact that anhedonic symptoms are reported in unaffected individuals with increased genetic risk for depression (see section on: *Familial association of anhedonia as a depressive endophenotype*), in combination with evidence that anhedonia may be a trait-like characteristic (see section on: *State-independence of anhedonia as a depressive endophenotype*). Collectively, these studies suggest that anhedonic symptoms may have predictive validity with regard to onset and severity of depression, poorer outcome, longer time to recovery, and higher likelihood of relapse.

The biological plausibility of anhedonia as a depressive endophenotype is supported by its association with dysfunctions of the brain reward system in neuroimaging studies [58–60]. Important brain areas involved in incentive processing include the dorsal striatum (e.g. caudate, putamen), the ventral striatum (e.g. nucleus accumbens), the anterior cingulate cortex (ACC), and the orbitofrontal cortex (OFC) [59,61,62]. As will be discussed below, neuroimaging studies promise to contribute to a more explicit understanding of which aspects of reward processing (e.g. hedonic coding, ability to link actions to rewards) are likely dysfunctional in depression, because (1) particular brain regions have been linked to specific facets of incentive processing (e.g. [63–68]); and (2) abnormal activation of these neural areas is evident in studies that directly assess reward processing in depression [60,69–74].

To begin with, the dorsal striatum (i.e. caudate, putamen) is important for coding reward prediction errors [64,75] and linking actions to rewards [76], and is strongly activated in response to unpredictable rewards [65]. Forbes and colleagues [74] recently reported that depressed adolescents exhibited lower caudate activation than psychiatrically healthy adolescents during monetary reward anticipation and outcome in a card-guessing task. Moreover, among the depressed adolescents, reduced caudate activation was associated with decreased subjective ratings of positive affect in real-world environments. Importantly, findings of lower caudate activation during reward anticipation and consumption in depressed adolescents are in line with similar results emerging from adult depressed samples (e.g. [60]). Specifically, utilizing fMRI and a monetary incentive delay task, we recently found that depressed adults displayed less bilateral caudate and left nucleus accumbens activation than controls during reward feedback and lower left putamen activation to reward-predicting cues [60]. The depressed participants also reported lower affective ratings during reward anticipation and consumption, and showed lower reward-related RT speeding. Accordingly, our results highlight depression-related impairment in functioning of both the dorsal and ventral striatum in response to a reward-processing task. Based on prior findings, we speculate that dysfunction in the dorsal and ventral striatum might index blunted action-reward reinforcement learning [76] and hedonic coding [67,77–79], respectively.

Reduced ventral striatal activation (nucleus accumbens) also emerged from a recent study conducted by Steele and colleagues [71], who utilized fMRI and a gambling task to examine postincentive behavioral adjustments and neural correlates in depression. Following positive feedback, participants with MDD failed to show the activation of ventral striatal regions and reduction in reaction time that was characteristic of controls, and the behavioral findings specifically correlated with anhedonic symptoms [71]. In a subsequent study, these investigators modeled reward prediction errors utilizing fMRI and a Pavlovian reward-learning paradigm that involved probabilistic associations between picture stimuli and water delivery to thirsty participants [73]. The authors found that treatment-resistant MDD participants, as compared to controls, had smaller reward-learning signals in the ventral striatum and dorsal ACC. Diminished ACC activation has also been observed in depressed children, relative to controls, during both the reward decision and reward outcome phases of a decision-making task [70]. Given that the ACC, especially its dorsal subdivision, has been implicated in linking outcome representations to actions and integrating reinforcement history to guide action [66], these findings suggest specific reward-related processes that may be impaired in depression.

In addition to the ACC, depressed children in the pediatric sample investigated by Forbes et al. [70] also exhibited lower activation than controls in the caudate and right OFC when receiving low-magnitude rewards. In light of prior findings, OFC dysfunction might index impairments in updating stimulus-reinforcement representations to guide behavior [63,80]. Taken as a whole, results from the aforementioned neuroimaging studies highlight certain aspects of reward processing that are likely to be dysfunctional in depression. For example, dysfunction in dorsal striatal regions, especially caudate hypoactivity, may reflect an impaired ability to learn connections between actions and rewards. Moreover, reduced functioning of the ventral striatal network (e.g. nucleus accumbens) in depression may be related to impaired hedonic coding and, along with dACC dysfunction, may underlie difficulty updating reward predictions. Of note, reduced ventral striatal activation in response to positive cues is largest in depressed individuals reporting elevated anhedonic symptoms [58,81], providing important convergent validity. Finally, OFC dysfunctions may be linked to impaired representation of the reward value of stimuli, as well as difficulty updating associations between stimuli and outcomes. Although the reviewed neuroimaging studies enhance our understanding of reward processing in depression, the aforementioned hypotheses need to be further examined using various paradigms in future studies before these theories can be definitively asserted.

Specificity of anhedonia as a depressive endophenotype

There is limited support for the specificity of anhedonia as a depressive endophenotype because the presence of anhedonia has been demonstrated in other mental illnesses, especially schizophrenia and substance use disorders [82,83]. In a recent examination of anhedonia in patients with depression, psychosis, or substance abuse, all three patient groups demonstrated significantly higher scores on a self-report measure of anhedonia, the Snaith–Hamilton Pleasure scale, relative to controls [84]; however, depressed patients also scored significantly higher than the two other patient groups. With regard to anhedonia in substance abusers, Martin-Soelch and colleagues [85] found that former opiate addicts, as compared to controls, showed reduced activation of neural reward circuits in response to non-monetary positive reinforcement. Although this neural hypoactivation in former opiate addicts did not extend to monetary positive reinforcement, their subjective ratings of monetary value were significantly lower than controls. Along with characterizing previous drug abusers, anhedonia may play a key role in relapse into drug use, likely due to reduced dopamine (DA) release associated with withdrawal [86]. However, the specific ways in which anhedonia and substance abuse are related, including the directionality between these factors, are complicated by comorbid psychopathology and remain to be fully elucidated.

In addition to its association with substance use disorders, anhedonia has also been closely linked to schizophrenia, and is indeed considered a prominent negative symptom of this disorder [87]. In a longitudinal study of schizophrenia and MDD, Blanchard and colleagues [88] found that both groups had higher scores than controls on a self-report measure of social anhedonia at baseline (inpatient hospitalization). Critically, whereas social anhedonic symptoms significantly declined in recovered depressed patients at a one-year follow-up, these symptoms remained stable in schizophrenia patients, raising the possibility that anhedonic symptoms may be trait-like in schizophrenia and more state-dependent in MDD. In an attempt to clarify the relationships between anhedonia, depression, and schizophrenia, Romney and Candido [89] used factor analysis to examine the loading of anhedonia on three main factors – depression, positive and negative symptoms of schizophrenia. Using self-report measures from schizophrenic and depressed samples, they reported that anhedonia loaded significantly on the depression factor but not the negative symptoms factor, and concluded that anhedonia is predominantly a depressive symptom that should be differentiated from the general affective blunting characteristic of schizophrenia. Conversely, as highlighted by Loas [90], other researchers who conducted related factor-analytic studies found anhedonic symptoms in schizophrenia to be independent of depressive symptoms (e.g. [91,92]). In another study relevant to this debate, Joiner and colleagues [93] found that MDD patients, as compared to schizophrenic patients, had significantly higher scores on the Beck Depression Inventory (BDI) anhedonic symptoms scale, while both groups had comparable non-anhedonic depressive symptoms scores and total BDI scores. These authors concluded that a much stronger relationship exists between anhedonic symptoms and depressive versus schizophrenic diagnostic status, lending support for anhedonia as a relatively specific marker for depression.

While the contrasting results of the aforementioned studies remain to be clarified, the use of "objective" laboratory-based measures of anhedonia may help to resolve some of the discrepancies by identifying specific aspects of reward processing that might be differentially affected in various clinical syndromes. In this regard, findings from recent studies by our laboratory [13] and Gold's group [94] provide initial evidence that different disorders might affect distinct aspects of reward processing. Of note, both studies used the same probabilistic reward task to evaluate how participants modulated their behavior as a function of reinforcement history. We found that unmedicated MDD patients had a reduced response bias toward the more frequently rewarded stimulus in the absence of immediate reward, although they were responsive to single rewards [13]. In contrast, Heerey, Bell-Warren and Gold [94] reported that participants with schizophrenia showed a normative response bias and did not have impaired sensitivity to reward or impaired ability to modulate behavior based on prior rewards received. Of note, these researchers also administered a probabilistic decision-making task to the same participants with schizophrenia and controls, and the schizophrenia group exhibited a reduced ability to evaluate potential outcomes when given competing response options, likely stemming from working memory deficits. Overall, Heerey, Bell-Warren and Gold [94] postulated that the fundamental mechanisms underlying reward-based learning in schizophrenia may actually be unimpaired, but these individuals might lack the ability to integrate such affective cues with other cognitive information to assess potential outcomes and guide behavior.[3] Accordingly, this initial evidence suggests that reward-related behavior in schizophrenia and MDD might be characterized by distinct dysfunctions.

Although anhedonic symptoms may not be exclusive to depression, some specificity to depression in relation to other mental illnesses, such as anxiety, has been demonstrated. Given the high degree of clinical overlap between depression and anxiety [97], much time

---

[3] It is of note that Heerey, Bell-Warren and Gold's [94] findings of unimpaired reward sensitivity in schizophrenia are limited by the fact that patients were medicated during testing and smoking status was not taken into account; the latter is a particularly relevant consideration since there are high rates of smoking in schizophrenia [95], and nicotine has been found to increase response bias in the same task used by Heerey and colleagues [96].

and effort has been expended towards parsing out which variables aid in differentiating between these illnesses. As suggested by a tripartite model of symptom clusters proposed by Watson and colleagues [98], although high negative affect characterizes both depression and anxiety, low positive affect is relatively specific to depression. Following from this model, various studies have demonstrated associations between depressive symptoms and reduced generation, recall, and anticipation of positive experiences that are not apparent in relation to anxiety symptoms [47,48,99,100].

For instance, MacLeod et al. [99] found that depressed patients, in contrast to patients with panic disorder or healthy controls, generated fewer positive experiences in response to various time-frame cues for both memory recall and future-thinking in a verbal fluency paradigm. In a subsequent study using a related paradigm, depressive symptoms – but not anxiety symptoms – were associated with a reduction in anticipated future positive experiences [47]. Similarly, Miranda and Mennin [48] reported that a greater propensity to predict that positive events would not happen in the future, and an increased level of certainty about these predictions, was associated with higher depression symptoms, but not anxiety symptoms. Finally, this pattern of results was extended to a pediatric sample of primary school children, in which probability ratings of self-referential future positive events were likewise negatively associated with levels of depression, but not levels of anxiety [100].

There is also evidence of specificity for depression over anxiety with respect to impaired perceptual processing of positively valenced cues and reduced ability to modify behavior as a function of rewards. First, individuals with MDD, as compared to individuals with social anxiety disorder and controls, have been shown to require a higher level of emotional expression in order to identify happy faces [40]. Second, utilizing a probabilistic reward task with a non-clinical sample, Pizzagalli, Jahn, and O'Shea [12] found that a reduced response bias toward a more frequently rewarded stimulus was specifically associated with anhedonic symptoms and not with symptoms of anxiety or general distress. These findings were replicated and extended in later studies using both non-clinical [101] and MDD [13] samples. Finally, in the abovementioned study by Forbes and colleagues [51], a reduced propensity to choose high-probability, high-reward options in a gambling task predicted depressive symptoms, but not anxiety symptoms, one year later. Collectively, the empirical evidence summarized in this section supports the notion that anhedonia symptoms are relatively specific to depression over anxiety.

State-independence of anhedonia as a depressive endophenotype

Relatively few studies in MDD samples have examined whether the symptoms of anhedonia reflect state or trait characteristics. Nevertheless, initial support for the temporal stability of anhedonia has emerged from investigations in which researchers have compared individuals who are actively experiencing clinical symptoms of depression with those who are in a remitted or recovered phase of the illness [43,102–104]. In the earliest of these studies, previously depressed patients retested during remission continued to demonstrate less frequent endorsement of positive words (non-depressed content adjectives), but not negative words (depressed content adjectives), than control subjects in a self-referent encoding task [102]. As suggested by the authors, these results raise the possibility that reduced positive self-image might represent a vulnerability factor for future depressive episodes. Ramel and colleagues [103] similarly found that remitted depressed participants, but not controls, recalled significantly fewer self-referent positive words following a sad mood induction compared to before the mood induction. The findings in remitted depressed individuals across both of these studies mirror the reduced endorsement and recall of self-referent positive words seen in currently depressed individuals [105]. In another experiment involving a negative mood induction, remitted subjects with a history of MDD were less likely than controls to associate themselves with happiness on an Implicit Association Test (IAT), irrespective of current mood state [104]. Along these lines, Joormann and Gotlib [43] reported that both currently and formerly depressed individuals failed to demonstrate a positive attentional bias towards happy faces that was characteristic of control participants during a dot-probe task. Interestingly, using a similar task combined with a sad mood induction, these researchers also found that unaffected children of depressed mothers failed to demonstrate an attentional bias towards happy faces [106]. Collectively, these findings demonstrate the existence or persistence of anhedonic symptoms (e.g. lower endorsement and recall of self-referential positive traits, and blunted attentional positivity biases) in fully remitted subjects and in other individuals at increased risk for depression. Accordingly, such results indicate that reduced positive self-image and blunted attentional biases toward incentive stimuli might increase vulnerability to depression and be state-independent.

Additional evidence of reduced reactivity to positive cues that continues beyond an active depressive episode comes from psychophysiological studies. For example, in an event-related potential (ERP) study by Nandrino and colleagues [107], first-episode depressed patients exhibited a reduction in P300 amplitude to positive words that was still present after treatment. Since the P300 is thought to index postidentification processes of discriminating and categorizing stimuli [108], these results may reflect state-independent hedonic processing deficits – specifically, impairment in the categorization of positive stimuli. In another electroencephalography (EEG) study, remitted depressed patients demonstrated reduced left-sided anterior resting EEG activity [109], mirroring patterns described in currently depressed patients [110]. Given that left prefrontal cortex activity has been associated with approach-related behaviors and appetitive goals [111,112], the findings of left-sided anterior hypoactivation across depressed and remitted individuals may reflect trait-like anhedonia.

However, it is important to note that not all studies lend credence to the notion of state-independence of anhedonic symptoms. For example, in the aforementioned study by Blanchard and colleagues [88], self-reported social anhedonia scores of depressed patients declined over a one-year follow-up in recovered patients, which suggests state dependence of social anhedonia in depression. A similar conclusion was drawn in a more recent study where individuals with current depression, but not those with remitted depression, reported diminished emotional responsiveness (i.e. lower self-reported ratings of happiness and enthusiasm) to anticipated reward, as compared to never depressed individuals [113]. One factor potentially contributing to both sets of results could be that experimental paradigms may need to include negative mood inductions to prime participants in order to see biased processing in a remitted depressed sample [114]. In a study that used such mood induction methods, results were mixed with respect to state-independence of anhedonic symptoms: both currently and remitted depressed youth recalled a significantly smaller amount of positive words than controls following a sad mood induction, but only currently depressed subjects exhibited a reduced endorsement of positive traits as well [115]. Accordingly, although there is some support for the temporal stability of anhedonia, further studies are necessary to determine whether specific components of anhedonia might persist after remission and be independent of illness status.

Familial association of anhedonia as a depressive endophenotype

In order to assess whether anhedonia fulfills the criterion of familial association, we turn to studies that have examined anhedonic symptoms in unaffected (e.g. no current or past diagnosis of mental disorder) first-degree relatives of patients with depression as compared to the general population. For example, Le Masurier and colleagues [116] reported that unaffected first-degree relatives of individuals with MDD took significantly longer to make self-referential categorizations of positive personality characteristics than age-matched controls; both groups were faster, however, to categorize positive than negative traits, suggesting a relatively reduced positive bias in the former group. Although a depressed comparison group was not included in this study, depressed patients were slower to identify positive words on a go/no-go task in an earlier study [117], indicating similarities in anhedonia-related information processing between individuals with depression and their unaffected relatives. A reduced positive bias has also been noted in never-disordered daughters of mothers with a history of recurrent MDD as compared to never-disordered daughters of mothers with no history of Axis I psychopathology [106]. In this study, a dot-probe task with emotional faces was administered to participants after a negative mood induction. The daughters of mothers with a history of depression failed to show the selective attention to positive facial expressions exhibited by the control daughters; rather, unlike controls, they displayed selective attention to negative facial expressions. Of note, the lack of positivity bias seen in the daughters of mothers with a history of depression was also found in both currently and formerly depressed patients by this same group of researchers using a similar dot-probe paradigm [43].

The mother–daughter findings by Joormann and colleagues complement a previous report on another pediatric sample with depressed versus non-depressed mothers [118]. In this earlier study, high-risk children endorsed significantly fewer positive words and recalled a higher proportion of endorsed negative words than low-risk children in a self-referent encoding task, but only following a negative mood induction. However, a notable strength of the more recent study by Joormann and colleagues [106] is that they obtained diagnostic information on the children and thus could rule out the possibility that current or past mental illness in their high-risk sample might have contributed to their results. In this way, assessment of individuals who have never expressed mental illness enables a more unambiguous deduction that observed findings may represent a vulnerability to depression rather than a consequence of psychopathology.

In a further study that took into account history of depression, Farmer and colleagues [119] utilized a sib-pair design and the Temperament and Character Inventory (TCI) to examine the familiality of various personality dimensions including reward dependence – a temperament trait reflecting domains such as social attachment, dependence on the approval of others, and sentimentality [120]. Of note, MDD patients tend to show reduced levels of reward dependence as compared to control individuals [121]. Interestingly, Farmer and colleagues found that never-depressed siblings of depressed probands had higher reward dependence scores than never-depressed siblings of healthy control probands. However, siblings of depressed probands with a history of depression themselves had lower reward dependence scores than either of these groups, indicating the possibility that high reward dependence may act as a protective factor against developing depression.

Finally, in the first fMRI study to compare asymptomatic juvenile offspring of parents with MDD to those of healthy parents, Monk and colleagues [122] found that high-risk offspring showed reduced nucleus accumbens activation when passively viewing happy faces (and increased nucleus accumbens activation when passively viewing fearful faces) relative to low-risk offspring. The neural responsiveness to positive stimuli found in the high-risk offspring parallels findings of reduced activation in the nucleus accumbens in response to happy faces [123] or reward feedback [60] in adults with MDD. Overall, empirical evidence that anhedonia-related emotional processing biases and reduced positivity biases occur more frequently in unaffected relatives of ill individuals than the general population lends support for the familial association of anhedonia as a depressive endophenotype, and suggests it may represent a risk factor for depression.

Heritability of anhedonia as a depressive endophenotype

Relatively few studies have examined the heritability of anhedonia (i.e. whether a proportion of its variance can be attributable to genetic variance), and some have investigated this topic in psychiatrically healthy samples or within the context of disorders other than MDD. In addition, the majority of such research has focused on self-report measures and only one study to date has used an objective behavioral measure of hedonic capacity, along with self-report measures, to investigate potential genetic contributions [124]. In this study, the same probabilistic reward task previously mentioned was administered to a small sample ($n = 70$; 35 twin pairs) of monozygotic (MZ) and dizygotic (DZ) twin pairs who reported no current or past psychiatric disorder. Model fitting revealed that 46% of the variance in hedonic capacity was accounted for by additive genetic factors, while 54% was accounted for by individual-specific environmental factors [124].

These results extend previous twin studies that have relied solely on self-report measures to assess the heritability of anhedonia. The earliest evidence of genetic influences on hedonic capacity comes from a study in a sample of college undergraduates by Dworkin and Saczynski [125], in which the intraclass correlation coefficients for a scale of hedonic capacity (items selected from the Minnesota Multiphasic Personality Inventory and the California Psychological Inventory) were significantly higher for MZ twin pairs (0.63) than DZ twin pairs (0.41). Subsequent twin studies similarly reported intraclass correlation coefficients that were significantly higher for MZ than DZ twin pairs (e.g. [126,127]), lending support for the notion that genetic factors contribute to the phenotypic expression of anhedonia. In one of these studies, at least one member of each twin pair had schizophrenia, and anhedonia levels were rated in a semistructured clinical interview [126]; the other study used an anhedonic subscale of a "schizotypy" Self-Report Questionnaire with a population-based twin registry [127]. Of note, an important limitation of these early studies is that they did not include model fitting on the variance-covariance matrices for MZ and DZ twin pairs to estimate the specific contributions of additive genetic, dominant genetic, common environment, and non-shared environment/measurement error.

In subsequent twin studies where investigators did perform such model fitting, heritability estimates of hedonic capacity range from 22% to 67% [128–135]. This broad range of heritability estimates might be partially accounted for by the fact that various self-report measures might be assessing different facets of hedonic capacity or have different psychometric characteristics (e.g. validity, reliability). Further research, including the evaluation of anhedonia across MZ and DZ twin pairs discordant for depression, and the utilization of objective measures of anhedonia in these samples, is necessary to obtain a more explicit understanding of heritability estimates for anhedonia. Nevertheless, results from twin studies to date suggest that genetic variance accounts for a considerable proportion of the variance in anhedonia. Importantly, given that heritability of MDD is estimated to be between 31% and 42% [136], heritability estimates for anhedonia may be even higher than those for MDD, which underscores a potential advantage of using an endophenotypic approach.

Cosegregation of anhedonia as a depressive endophenotype

There is a notable lack of studies investigating anhedonia across affected and unaffected relatives of depressed individuals. However, in the aforementioned sib-pair study conducted by Farmer and colleagues [119], siblings of depressed individuals who had a history of depression themselves had significantly lower reward dependence scores compared with never-depressed siblings of depressed individuals. Results from this study support the notion that within families of depressed individuals, anhedonia may occur more frequently in family members who are affected with the illness than in family members who are unaffected by the illness. Nevertheless, additional studies are clearly needed to further investigate the cosegregation of anhedonia.

Current directions in objective laboratory measurements of anhedonia

Given that self-report measures of anhedonic symptoms are inherently subjective and vulnerable to reporting biases, the development of more objective measures of anhedonia is well warranted. As a first step in this direction, our laboratory recently developed a probabilistic reward task to provide an objective measure of reward responsiveness [12]. The task, which was adapted from a prior paradigm described by Tripp and Alsop [137], involves a differential reinforcement schedule to obtain an objective measurement of an individual's ability to adapt behavior as a function of reinforcement history [12]. In this task, participants are briefly presented with one of two stimuli and asked to determine which stimulus appeared on a computer screen. Importantly, the two stimuli are physically very similar and presented very briefly (100 ms), making the differentiation quite difficult. Critically, unbeknownst to the participants, correct identification of one stimulus is followed by reward feedback (e.g. "Correct!! You won 5 cents!") three times more frequently than correct identification of the other stimulus. Under this experimental setting, healthy subjects quickly develop a robust response bias toward the more frequently rewarded stimulus [12,137,138]. Notably, the probabilistic nature of the task prevents participants from being able to use the outcome of a single trial to deduce which stimulus is more profitable; rather, participants must integrate reinforcement history over time to perform most successfully on the task.

Importantly, based on results from initial studies, the psychometric properties of this task appear promising. For example, in two separate studies, the test–retest reliability for response bias over approximately 38 days was 0.56–0.57 [12,139]. Moreover, as mentioned above, the heritability of reward responsiveness in a twin study using this task was estimated to be approximately 48% [124]. Furthermore, studies utilizing the probabilistic reward task with participants presumed to be impaired in reinforcement learning – such as individuals with affective disorders [7,140] – provide evidence of construct validity. A reduced response bias towards the more frequently rewarded stimulus has been described in unmedicated patients with MDD [13], medicated euthymic patients with bipolar disorder [141], and students with elevated depressive symptoms [12]. In the study with unmedicated MDD patients, trial-by-trial probability analyses indicated that this group had a reduced response bias toward the more frequently rewarded stimulus in the absence of immediate reward, but was responsive to single rewards. Moreover, as noted earlier, this dysfunction was correlated with anhedonic symptoms ($r = 0.52$, $p < 0.05$) and not with symptoms of anxiety or general distress.

Importantly, performance on the probabilistic reward task is also associated with activation of reward-related neural regions, in particular the dACC and caudate. Participants who fail to develop a response bias towards the more frequently rewarded stimulus have been found to show significantly lower activation in caudate and dACC regions in response to reward feedback than those who develop such a response bias [139]. Furthermore, activation of dACC regions specifically correlates with this learning ability ($r = 0.40$, $p < 0.03$). These findings are in line with previous studies that have demonstrated a link between dACC region activation and the ability to integrate reinforcement history over time (e.g. [66]) as well as studies implicating the caudate in learning action-reward contingencies (e.g. [76]).

Finally, given that DA is believed to play a key role in reward-related learning [142], two studies have been conducted to examine whether pharmacological manipulations affecting DA either indirectly [96] or directly [143] would influence development of response bias in the probabilistic reward task. In the first case, healthy non-smokers were administered a single dose of transdermal nicotine (7–14 mg) in a randomized, double-blind, placebo-controlled crossover design; nicotine was found to increase response bias towards the more frequently rewarded stimulus [96]. Further studies will be needed to determine whether the mechanisms underlying these findings are similar to those emerging from animal studies, in which nicotine activates the presynaptic nicotinic receptors on mesocorticolimbic DA neurons to increase appetitive responding [144]. In the second case, healthy participants who received a single 0.5 mg dose of the D2/3 agonist pramipexole 2 h prior to completing the probabilistic reward task demonstrated impaired reinforcement learning as compared to those who received placebo [143]. Here again, future studies are necessary to explore whether the mechanisms underlying these findings emulate related animal data [145] and reflect pramipexole-induced activation of DA autoreceptors and corresponding reductions in phasic DA bursts. In spite of the need for studies directly assessing DA signaling in humans, it is important to emphasize that impaired reinforcement learning in the pramipexole group could be simulated by decreased reward-related presynaptic DA signaling in a neural network model of striato-cortical function in subsequent analyses of this data set [146]. In sum, evidence supports the psychometric properties of the probabilistic reward task, and accordingly, its potential usefulness to objectively measure specific reward-related dysfunctions.

Summary and future directions

The overarching goal of this chapter was to review human literature pointing to the potential utility of applying an endophenotypic approach to depression research. In doing so, we specifically focused on anhedonia, which is emerging as one of the most promising endophenotypes of depression (e.g. [7,12,13]). In line with this conceptualization, we discussed empirical evidence suggesting that anhedonia meets the criteria of biological and clinical plausibility, familial association, and heritability; mixed or limited findings exist for state-independence and specificity, and few studies have addressed cosegregation.

The research presented in this chapter supports a strong relationship between anhedonia and depression from both clinical and biological viewpoints. In particular, individuals with depression are characterized by reduced affective and behavioral reactivity to positive stimuli (highlighting possible encoding dysfunctions) and impaired abilities to use reinforcement history to modify behavior, which might be linked to difficulties in estimating the occurrence of past positive events and predicting future positive events. Although conclusive statements would be premature, it is likely that such behavioral impairments are linked to dysfunctions in reward-related neural regions, including the dorsal and ventral striatum, the ACC, and the OFC. Importantly, anhedonic symptoms and behavior have predictive value in determining depression onset, course, time to recovery, and likelihood of relapse. As a corpus, these findings underscore the role of anhedonia in the emergence, maintenance, and exacerbation of depression.

Although anhedonia is not exclusive to depression, it is specific to depression over anxiety, which is an important consideration given the high rates of comorbidity between these disorders [97]. Moreover, there is evidence to suggest that symptoms of anhedonia may be relatively stable over time (e.g. outside of depressive episodes), and are present to a greater degree in the unaffected relatives of depressed individuals than the general population, which lends credence to the notion that anhedonia may be a vulnerability factor in the development of depression. Finally, given that heritability estimates for anhedonia might exceed those for depression, it is plausible that investigations focused on anhedonia may enable us to get closer to pinpointing some of the genes that contribute to an increased risk for depression. Recent findings that specific DA-coding polymorphisms affect activation within the brain reward pathway (e.g. [147–149]) highlight promising targets for future investigations of the genetic underpinnings of anhedonia.

There are many additional avenues for future research that promise to provide a more comprehensive understanding of anhedonia as a depressive endophenotype. First, additional neuroimaging studies are needed to build upon prior findings of associations between various aspects of reward processing (e.g. reward anticipation vs. consumption) and dysfunctions of specific reward-related neural circuitry [58,60]. Second, in light of the well-documented link between stress and depression (e.g. [150]), and initial evidence that anhedonia may serve as a central bridge connecting them [101,151–153], further investigations characterizing the relationship and underlying mechanisms between stress and anhedonia are warranted. Third, in order to more fully address the endophenotypic criteria of heritability and cosegregation, there is a critical need for studies that investigate anhedonia across MZ and DZ twin pairs discordant for depression, and across affected and unaffected relatives of depressed individuals. In particular, studies assessing MZ twin pairs discordant for depression may help to clarify whether anhedonia is a vulnerability factor for the development of depression or a consequence of the disorder. Along similar lines, studies focusing on individuals at risk for depression (e.g. children or siblings of depressed probands) before the onset of a first major depressive episode will be required to elucidate whether anhedonia and related neural dysfunctions are a risk factor for depression or an epiphenomenon of the illness. Fourth, in light of differences in the phenomenology of depression between children and adults [154], as well as gender differences in the epidemiology of depression [155], there is a critical need for research that will examine the developmental trajectory of anhedonia over the lifespan and associated gender differences.

Across all of these lines of inquiry, the use of objective measures of anhedonia (such as the probabilistic reward task described in this chapter), and mathematical modeling of reward prediction errors (e.g. [71,73]), may be beneficial to identify the extent and nature of anhedonic deficits precisely. Finally, in the spirit of moving towards personalized treatment in psychopathology [156], it will be important to determine whether individuals characterized by specific behavioral or neural anhedonic phenotypes might be particularly responsive to cognitive and/or behavioral treatments centered on positive reinforcement (e.g. [157,158]), or pharmacological interventions targeting dopaminergic dysfunctions (e.g. [159]). Ultimately, it is hoped that taking an endophenotypic approach will help us to elucidate the etiological pathways underlying depression, leading to improvements in the validity of our classification system and, more importantly, to increased effectiveness of treatment and prevention methods.

References

1. Moussavi, S., Chatterji, S., Verdes, E., Tandon, A., Patel, V., and Ustun, B. 2007, *Lancet*, **370**, 851.

2. Kessler, R. C., Berglund, P., Demler, O., et al. 2003, *J. Am. Med. Assoc.*, **289**, 3095.

3. Kessler, R. C., Berglund, P., Demler, O., Jin, R., Merikangas, K. R., and Walters, E. E. 2005, *Arch. Gen. Psychiatry*, **62**, 593.

4. Merikangas, K. R., Ames, M., Cui, L., et al. 2007, *Arch. Gen. Psychiatry*, **64**, 1180.

5. Kessler, R. C., and Wang, P. S. 2009, *Handbook of Depression*, I. H. Gotlib and C. L. Hammen (Eds.), New York, Guilford Press, 5.

6. Warden, D., Rush, A. J., Trivedi, M. H., Fava, M., and Wisniewski, S. R. 2007, *Curr. Psychiatry Rep.*, **9**, 449.

7. Hasler, G., Drevets, W. C., Manji, H. K., and Charney, D. S. 2004, *Neuropsychopharmacology*, **29**, 1765.

8. Meyer-Lindenberg, A., and Weinberger, D. R. 2006, *Nat. Rev. Neurosci.*, **7**, 818.

9. Hyman, S. E. 2007, *Nat. Rev. Neurosci.*, **8**, 725.

10. Gottesman, I. I., and Gould, T. D. 2003, *Am. J. Psychiatry*, **160**, 636.

11. American Psychiatric Association. 2000, *Diagnostic and Statistical Manual of Mental Disorders*, 4th edn., text revision, Washington, DC, American Psychiatric Press.

12. Pizzagalli, D. A., Jahn, A. L., and O'Shea, J. P. 2005, *Biol. Psychiatry*, **57**, 319.

13. Pizzagalli, D. A., Iosifescu, D., Hallett, L. A., Ratner, K. G., and Fava, M. 2009, *J. Psychiatr. Res.*, **43**, 76.

14. Luyten, P., and Blatt, S. J. 2007, *Psychiatry*, **70**, 85.

15. Hasler, G., Drevets, W. C., Gould, T. D., Gottesman, I. I., and Manji, H. K. 2006, *Biol. Psychiatry*, **60**, 93.

16. Merikangas, K. R., and Swendsen, J. D. 1997, *Epidemiol. Rev.*, **19**, 144.

17. Uher, R. 2008, *Mol. Psychiatry*, **13**, 1070.

18. Flint, J., and Munafo, M. R. 2007, *Psychol. Med.*, **37**, 163.

19. Gershon, E. S., and Goldin, L. R. 1986, *Acta Psychiatr. Scand.*, **74**, 113.

20. Tsuang, M. T., Faraone, S. V., and Lyons, M. J. 1993, *Eur. Arch. Psychiatry Clin. Neurosci.*, **243**, 131.

21. Meehl, P. E. 1975, *Bull. Menninger Clin.*, **39**, 295.

22. Klein, D. F. 1987, *Anhedonia and Affect Deficit States*, D. C. Clark and J. Fawcett (Eds.), New York, PMA Publishing Corporation, 1.

23. Loas, G. 1996, *J. Affect. Disord.*, **41**, 39.

24. Berenbaum, H., and Oltmanns, T. F. 1992, *J. Abnorm. Psychol.*, **101**, 37.

25. Sloan, D. M., Strauss, M. E., and Wisner, K. L. 2001, *J. Abnorm. Psychol.*, **110**, 488.

26. Gehricke, J., and Shapiro, D. 2000, *Psychiatry Res.*, **95**, 157.

27. Renneberg, B., Heyn, K., Gebhard, R., and Bachmann, S. 2005, *J. Behav. Ther. Exp. Psychiatry*, **36**, 183.

28. Allen, N. B., Trinder, J., and Brennan, C. 1999, *Biol. Psychiatry*, **46**, 542.

29. Dunn, B. D., Dalgleish, T., Lawrence, A. D., Cusack, R., and Ogilvie, A. D. 2004, *J. Abnorm. Psychol.*, **113**, 654.

30. Kaviani, H., Gray, J. A., Checkley, S. A., Raven, P. W., Wilson, G. D., and Kumari, V. 2004, *J. Affect. Disord.*, **83**, 21.

31. Siegle, G. J., Thompson, W., Carter, C. S., Steinhauer, S. R., and Thase, M. E. 2007, *Biol. Psychiatry*, **61**, 198.

32. Chentsova-Dutton, Y. E., Chu, J. P., Tsai, J. L., Rottenberg, J., Gross, J. J., and Gotlib, I. H. 2007, *J. Abnorm. Psychol.*, **116**, 776.

33. Dichter, G. S., and Tomarken, A. J. 2008, *J. Abnorm. Psychol.*, **117**, 1.

34. Kan, Y., Mimura, M., Kamijima, K., and Kawamura, M. 2004, *J. Neurol. Neurosurg. Psychiatry*, **75**, 1667.

35. Leppanen, J. M., Milders, M., Bell, J. S., Terriere, E., and Hietanen, J. K. 2004, *Psychiatry Res.*, **128**, 123.

36. Merens, W., Booij, L., and Van Der Does, A. J. 2008, *Depress. Anxiety*, **25**, E27.

37. Mikhailova, E. S., Vladimirova, T. V., Iznak, A. F., Tsusulkovskaya, E. J., and Sushko, N. V. 1996, *Biol. Psychiatry*, **40**, 697.

38. Surguladze, S. A., Young, A. W., Senior, C., Brebion, G., Travis, M. J., and Phillips, M. L. 2004, *Neuropsychology*, **18**, 212.

39. Suslow, T., Junghanns, K., and Arolt, V. 2001, *Percept. Mot. Skills*, **92**, 857.

40. Joormann, J., and Gotlib, I. H. 2006, *J. Abnorm. Psychol.*, **115**, 705.

41. Kakolewski, K. E., Crowson, J. J., Jr., Sewell, K. W., and Cromwell, R. L. 1999, *Int. J. Psychophysiol.*, **34**, 283.

42. Wang, C. E., Brennen, T., and Holte, A. 2006, *Scand. J. Psychol.*, **47**, 505.

43. Joormann, J., and Gotlib, I. H. 2007, *J. Abnorm. Psychol.*, **116**, 80.

44. Karparova, S. P., Kersting, A., and Suslow, T. 2007, *Scand. J. Psychol.*, **48**, 1.

45. Buchwald, A. M. 1977, *J. Abnorm. Psychol.*, **86**, 443.

46. Nelson, R. E., and Craighead, W. E. 1977, *J. Abnorm. Psychol.*, **86**, 379.

47. MacLeod, A. K., and Salaminiou, E. 2001, *Cogn. Emot.*, **15**, 99.

48. Miranda, R., and Mennin, D. S. 2007, *Cogn. Ther. Res.*, **31**, 71.

49. Henriques, J. B., Glowacki, J. M., and Davidson, R. J. 1994, *J. Abnorm. Psychol.*, **103**, 460.

50. Henriques, J. B., and Davidson, R. 2000, *Cogn. Emot.*, **14**, 711.

51. Forbes, E. E., Shaw, D. S., and Dahl, R. E. 2007, *Biol. Psychiatry*, **61**, 633.

52. Williams, J. M. G., Watts, F. N., MacLeod, C., and Mathews, A. 1997, *Cognitive Psychology and Emotional Disorders*, 2nd edn., Chichester, Wiley.

53. Kasch, K. L., Rottenberg, J., Arnow, B. A., and Gotlib, I. H. 2002, *J. Abnorm. Psychol.*, **111**, 589.

54. McFarland, B. R., Shankman, S. A., Tenke, C. E., Bruder, G. E., and Klein, D. N. 2006, *J. Affect. Disord.*, **91**, 229.

55. Rottenberg, J., Kasch, K. L., Gross, J. J., and Gotlib, I. H. 2002, *Emotion*, **2**, 135.

56. Johnson, S. L., Joormann, J., and Gotlib, I. H. 2007, *Emotion*, **7**, 201.

57. Lethbridge, R., and Allen, N. B. 2008, *Behav. Res. Ther.*, **46**, 1142.

58. Keedwell, P. A., Andrew, C., Williams, S. C., Brammer, M. J., and Phillips, M. L. 2005, *Biol. Psychiatry*, **58**, 843.

59. Pizzagalli, D. A., Dillon, D. G., Bogdan, R., and Holmes, A. In press, *Neuroscience of Decision Making*, O. Vartanian, and D. Mandel (Eds.), New York, NY, Psychology Press.

60. Pizzagalli, D. A., Holmes, A. J., Dillon, D. G., et al. 2009, *Am. J. Psychiatry*, **166**, 702–10.

61. O'Doherty, J. P. 2004, *Curr. Opin. Neurobiol.*, **14**, 769.

62. Diekhof, E. K., Falkai, P., and Gruber, O. 2008, *Brain Res. Rev.*, **59**, 164.

63. Gottfried, J. A., O'Doherty, J., and Dolan, R. J. 2003, *Science*, **301**, 1104.

64. McClure, S. M., Berns, G. S., and Montague, P. R. 2003, *Neuron*, **38**, 339.

65. Tricomi, E. M., Delgado, M. R., and Fiez, J. A. 2004, *Neuron*, **41**, 281.

66. Rushworth, M. F., Behrens, T. E., Rudebeck, P. H., and Walton, M. E. 2007, *Trends Cogn. Sci.*, **11**, 168.

67. Wrase, J., Kahnt, T., Schlagenhauf, F., et al. 2007, *Neuroimage*, **36**, 1253.

68. Dillon, D. G., Holmes, A. J., Jahn, A. L., Bogdan, R., Wald, L. L., and Pizzagalli, D. A. 2008, *Psychophysiology*, **45**, 36.

69. Tremblay, L. K., Naranjo, C. A., Graham, S. J., et al. 2005, *Arch. Gen. Psychiatry*, **62**, 1228.

70. Forbes, E. E., Christopher May, J., Siegle, G. J., et al. 2006, *J. Child Psychol. Psychiatry*, **47**, 1031.

71. Steele, J. D., Kumar, P., and Ebmeier, K. P. 2007, *Brain*, **130**, 2367.

72. Knutson, B., Bhanji, J. P., Cooney, R. E., Atlas, L. Y., and Gotlib, I. H. 2008, *Biol. Psychiatry*, **63**, 686.

73. Kumar, P., Waiter, G., Ahearn, T., Milders, M., Reid, I., and Steele, J. D. 2008, *Brain*, **131**, 2084.

74. Forbes, E. E., Hariri, A. R., Martin, S. L., et al. 2009, *Am. J. Psychiatry*, **166**, 64.

75. O'Doherty, J. P., Dayan, P., Friston, K., Critchley, H., and Dolan, R. J. 2003, *Neuron*, **38**, 329.

76. Delgado, M. R. 2007, *Ann. NY Acad. Sci.*, **1104**, 70.

77. Delgado, M. R., Locke, H. M., Stenger, V. A., and Fiez, J. A. 2003, *Cogn. Affect. Behav. Neurosci.*, **3**, 27.

78. Knutson, B., Fong, G. W., Bennett, S. M., Adams, C. M., and Hommer, D. 2003, *Neuroimage*, **18**, 263.

79. Galvan, A., Hare, T. A., Davidson, M., Spicer, J., Glover, G., and Casey, B. J. 2005, *J. Neurosci.*, **25**, 8650.

80. Holland, P. C., and Gallagher, M. 2004, *Curr. Opin. Neurobiol.*, **14**, 148.

81. Epstein, J., Pan, H., Kocsis, J. H., et al. 2006, *Am. J. Psychiatry*, **163**, 1784.

82. Heinz, A., Schmidt, L. G., and Reischies, F. M. 1994, *Pharmacopsychiatry*, **27** Suppl 1, 7.

83. Horan, W. P., Kring, A. M., and Blanchard, J. J. 2006, *Schizophr. Bull.*, **32**, 259.

84. Franken, I. H., Rassin, E., and Muris, P. 2007, *J. Affect. Disord.*, **99**, 83.

85. Martin-Soelch, C., Chevalley, A. F., Kunig, G., et al. 2001, *Eur. J. Neurosci.*, **14**, 1360.

86. Volkow, N. D., Fowler, J. S., Wang, G. J., and Goldstein, R. Z. 2002, *Neurobiol. Learn. Mem.*, **78**, 610.

87. Andreasen, N. C., and Olsen, S. 1982, *Arch. Gen. Psychiatry*, **39**, 789.

88. Blanchard, J. J., Horan, W. P., and Brown, S. A. 2001, *J. Abnorm. Psychol.*, **110**, 363.

89. Romney, D. M., and Candido, C. L. 2001, *J. Nerv. Ment. Dis.*, **189**, 735.

90. Loas, G. 2002, *J. Nerv. Ment. Dis.*, **190**, 717.

91. Kitamura, T., and Suga, R. 1991, *Compr. Psychiatry*, **32**, 88.

92. Katsanis, J., Iacono, W. G., Beiser, M., and Lacey, L. 1992, *J. Abnorm. Psychol.*, **101**, 184.

93. Joiner, T. E., Brown, J. S., and Metalsky, G. I. 2003, *Psychiatry Res.*, **119**, 243.

94. Heerey, E. A., Bell-Warren, K. R., and Gold, J. M. 2008, *Biol. Psychiatry*, **64**, 62.

95. Kumari, V., and Postma, P. 2005, *Neurosci. Biobehav. Rev.*, **29**, 1021.

96. Barr, R. S., Pizzagalli, D. A., Culhane, M. A., Goff, D. C., and Evins, A. E. 2008, *Biol. Psychiatry*, **63**, 1061.

97. Kessler, R. C., Chiu, W. T., Demler, O., Merikangas, K. R., and Walters, E. E. 2005, *Arch. Gen. Psychiatry*, **62**, 617.

98. Watson, D., Weber, K., Assenheimer, J. S., Clark, L. A., Strauss, M. E., and McCormick, R. A. 1995, *J. Abnorm. Psychol.*, **104**, 3.

99. MacLeod, A. K., Tata, P., Kentish, J., and Jacobsen, H. 1997, *Cogn. Emot.*, **11**, 467.

100. Muris, P., and van der Heiden, S. 2006, *J. Anxiety Disord.*, **20**, 252.

101. Bogdan, R., and Pizzagalli, D. A. 2006, *Biol. Psychiatry*, **60**, 1147.

102. Dobson, K. S., and Shaw, B. F. 1987, *J. Abnorm. Psychol.*, **96**, 34.

103. Ramel, W., Goldin, P. R., Eyler, L. T., Brown, G. G., Gotlib, I. H., and McQuaid, J. R. 2007, *Biol. Psychiatry*, **61**, 231.

104. Meites, T. M., Deveney, C. M., Steele, K. T., Holmes, A. J., and Pizzagalli, D. A. 2008, *Behav. Res. Ther.*, **46**, 1078.

105. Gotlib, I. H., Kasch, K. L., Traill, S., Joormann, J., Arnow, B. A., and Johnson, S. L. 2004, *J. Abnorm. Psychol.*, **113**, 386.

106. Joormann, J., Talbot, L., and Gotlib, I. H. 2007, *J. Abnorm. Psychol.*, **116**, 135.

107. Nandrino, J. L., Dodin, V., Martin, P., and Henniaux, M. 2004, *J. Psychiatr. Res.*, **38**, 475.

108. Dien, J., Spencer, K. M., and Donchin, E. 2004, *Psychophysiology*, **41**, 665.

109. Henriques, J. B., and Davidson, R. J. 1990, *J. Abnorm. Psychol.*, **99**, 22.

110. Henriques, J. B., and Davidson, R. J. 1991, *J. Abnorm. Psychol.*, **100**, 535.

111. Davidson, R. J., Jackson, D. C., and Kalin, N. H. 2000, *Psychol. Bull.*, **126**, 890.

112. Pizzagalli, D. A., Sherwood, R. J., Henriques, J. B., and Davidson, R. J. 2005, *Psychol. Sci.*, **16**, 805.

113. McFarland, B. R., and Klein, D. N. 2009, *Depress. Anxiety*, **26**, 117.

114. Scher, C. D., Ingram, R. E., and Segal, Z. V. 2005, *Clin. Psychol. Rev.*, **25**, 487.

115. Timbremont, B., and Braet, C. 2004, *Behav. Res. Ther.*, **42**, 423.

116. Le Masurier, M., Cowen, P. J., and Harmer, C. J. 2007, *Psychol. Med.*, **37**, 403.

117. Murphy, F. C., Sahakian, B. J., Rubinsztein, J. S., et al. 1999, *Psychol. Med.*, **29**, 1307.

118. Taylor, L., and Ingram, R. E. 1999, *J. Abnorm. Psychol.*, **108**, 202.

119. Farmer, A., Mahmood, A., Redman, K., Harris, T., Sadler, S., and McGuffin, P. 2003, *Arch. Gen. Psychiatry*, **60**, 490.

120. Cloninger, C. R., Svrakic, D. M., and Przybeck, T. R. 1993, *Arch. Gen. Psychiatry*, **50**, 975.

121. Nery, F. G., Hatch, J. P., Nicoletti, M. A., et al. 2009, *Depress. Anxiety*, **26**, 382.

122. Monk, C. S., Klein, R. G., Telzer, E. H., et al. 2008, *Am. J. Psychiatry*, **165**, 90.

123. Surguladze, S., Brammer, M. J., Keedwell, P., et al. 2005, *Biol. Psychiatry*, **57**, 201.

124. Bogdan, R., and Pizzagalli, D. A. 2009, *Psychol. Med.*, **39**, 211.

125. Dworkin, R. H., and Saczynski, K. 1984, *J. Pers. Assess.*, **48**, 620.

126. Berenbaum, H., Oltmanns, T. F., and Gottesman, I. I. 1990, *Psychol. Med.*, **20**, 367.

127. Kendler, K. S., Ochs, A. L., Gorman, A. M., Hewitt, J. K., Ross, D. E., and Mirsky, A. F. 1991, *Psychiatry Res.*, **36**, 19.

128. Kendler, K. S., and Hewitt, J. 1992, *J. Pers. Disord.*, **6**, 1.

129. Heath, A. C., Cloninger, C. R., and Martin, N. G. 1994, *J. Pers. Soc. Psychol.*, **66**, 762.

130. Hay, D. A., Martin, N. G., Foley, D., Treloar, S. A., Kirk, K. M., and Heath, A. C. 2001, *Twin Res.*, **4**, 30.

131. MacDonald, A. W., 3rd, Pogue-Geile, M. F., Debski, T. T., and Manuck, S. 2001, *Schizophr. Bull.*, **27**, 47.

132. Ono, Y., Ando, J., Yoshimura, K., Momose, T., Hirano, M., and Kanba, S. 2002, *Mol. Psychiatry*, **7**, 948.

133. Linney, Y. M., Murray, R. M., Peters, E. R., MacDonald, A. M., Rijsdijk, F., and Sham, P. C. 2003, *Psychol. Med.*, **33**, 803.

134. Jang, K. L., Livesley, W. J., Taylor, S., Stein, M. B., and Moon, E. C. 2004, *J. Affect. Disord.*, **80**, 125.

135. Keller, M. C., and Nesse, R. M. 2005, *J. Affect. Disord.*, **86**, 27.

136. Sullivan, P. F., Neale, M. C., and Kendler, K. S. 2000, *Am. J. Psychiatry*, **157**, 1552.

137. Tripp, G., and Alsop, B. 1999, *J. Clin. Child. Psychol.*, **28**, 366.

138. McCarthy, D., and Davison, M. 1979, *J. Exp. Anal. Behav.*, **32**, 373.

139. Santesso, D. L., Dillon, D. G., Birk, J. L., et al. 2008, *Neuroimage*, **42**, 807.

140. Leibenluft, E., Charney, D. S., and Pine, D. S. 2003, *Biol. Psychiatry*, **53**, 1009.

141. Pizzagalli, D. A., Goetz, E., Ostacher, M., Iosifescu, D. V., and Perlis, R. H. 2008, *Biol. Psychiatry*, **64**, 162.

142. Dunlop, B. W., and Nemeroff, C. B. 2007, *Arch. Gen. Psychiatry*, **64**, 327.

143. Pizzagalli, D. A., Evins, A. E., Schetter, E. C., et al. 2008, *Psychopharmacology*, **196**, 221.

144. Kenny, P. J., and Markou, A. 2006, *Neuropsychopharmacology*, **31**, 1203.

145. Piercey, M. F., Hoffmann, W. E., Smith, M. W., and Hyslop, D. K. 1996, *Eur. J. Pharmacol.*, **312**, 35.

146. Santesso, D. L., Evins, A. E., Frank, M. J., Schetter, E. C., Bogdan, R., and Pizzagalli, D. A. 2009, *Hum. Brain Mapp.*, **30**, 1963.

147. Yacubian, J., Sommer, T., Schroeder, K., et al. 2007, *Proc. Natl Acad. Sci. USA*, **104**, 8125.

148. Dreher, J. C., Kohn, P., Kolachana, B., Weinberger, D. R., and Berman, K. F. 2009, *Proc. Natl Acad. Sci. USA*, **106**, 617.

149. Forbes, E. E., Brown, S. M., Kimak, M., Ferrell, R. E., Manuck, S. B., and Hariri, A. R. 2009, *Mol. Psychiatry*, **14**, 60.

150. Hammen, C. 2005, *Annu. Rev. Clin. Psychol.*, **1**, 293.

151. Berenbaum, H., and Connelly, J. 1993, *J. Abnorm. Psychol.*, **102**, 474.

152. Anisman, H., and Matheson, K. 2005, *Neurosci. Biobehav. Rev.*, **29**, 525.

153. Pizzagalli, D. A., Bogdan, R., Ratner, K. G., and Jahn, A. L. 2007, *Behav. Res. Ther.*, **45**, 2742.

154. Garber, J., Gallerani, C. M., and Frankel, S. A. 2009, *Handbook of Depression*, I. H. Gotlib, and C. L. Hammen (Eds.), New York, Guilford Press, 405.

155. Nolen-Hoeksema, S., and Hilt, L. M. 2009, *Handbook of Depression*, I. H. Gotlib, and C. L. Hammen (Eds.), New York, Guilford, 386.

156. Insel, T. R. 2009, *Arch. Gen. Psychiatry*, **66**, 128.

157. Dimidjian, S., Hollon, S. D., Dobson, K. S., et al. 2006, *J. Consult. Clin. Psychol.*, **74**, 658.

158. Ekers, D., Richards, D., and Gilbody, S. 2008, *Psychol. Med.*, **38**, 611.

159. Corrigan, M. H., Denahan, A. Q., Wright, C. E., Ragual, R. J., and Evans, D. L. 2000, *Depress. Anxiety*, **11**, 58.

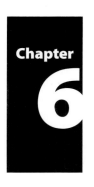

Chapter 6

Genetic and genomic studies of major depressive disorder

Roy H. Perlis

Abstract

Family studies indicate that major depressive disorder runs in families, although family members' risk for other psychiatric disorders may also be increased. Twin and adoption studies suggest that about one-third of the liability for MDD is inherited. Studies investigating individual candidate genes have failed to implicate any single gene in MDD risk. Emerging evidence from genome-wide association studies may identify novel risk genes, although any individual genetic variation appears likely to have only modest effect. Whether focusing on clinical subtypes of MDD, or relying on imaging or other biomarkers rather than clinical features, will expedite the process of gene discovery remains to be determined.

Introduction

Questioning about a family history of psychiatric illness is part of a standard clinical assessment in psychiatry. Clinicians as well as patients appear to recognize that illnesses such as depression, like cardiac disease or diabetes, appear to "run in families." Indeed, studies spanning more than 25 years, using a variety of designs, support this notion. In this chapter, we review studies which have examined aspects of the genetic epidemiology of MDD. We begin with the studies which have attempted to characterize familiality, then those which estimate heritability, the extent to which such familiality may be explained by genetic rather than environmental features. We next discuss efforts to find regions of the genome which may account for this inherited risk, exploring reasons why such efforts to date have yielded limited results. Finally, we explore possible novel directions in gene-finding in MDD.

Does MDD run in families?

Typically, the first question in investigating the genetic basis of disease is determining whether that disease is more common in some families than in others. Typically such studies begin by identifying a patient with MDD (the proband), and matching that patient with a 'control' individual without MDD. By assessing the family members of the proband and the control, it is then possible to compare the magnitude of risk for MDD in family members of the proband to risk for MDD in family members of the control subject. Thus, in essence the family study is a kind of case-control study [1].

In considering these kinds of studies, a number of features bear consideration. First, how were the patients identified and matched with controls? If these two groups are not well-matched, the estimates of risk may be falsely elevated. For example, because socioeconomic

Next Generation Antidepressants: Moving Beyond Monoamines to Discover Novel Treatment Strategies for Mood Disorders, ed. Chad E. Beyer and Stephen M. Stahl. Published by Cambridge University Press.
© Cambridge University Press 2010.

status (SES) may be a risk for MDD, if the control group is drawn from a higher SES, their risk of MDD may be decreased. Second, how was MDD diagnosed? The optimal assessment employs clinical interview of the family members directly. However, in many cases this is not practical: family members may be deceased, distant from the study site, or unwilling to participate in the study. Therefore, some studies employ indirect interview, in which the proband (or other family members) are asked to describe the individuals who cannot be interviewed. A potential problem with this approach is analogous to recall bias: family members may be more likely to recognize or infer MDD (or other psychiatric disorders) knowing that the proband is ill. The clinical equivalent of this phenomenon is the patient, newly diagnosed with MDD, who reports "now that I think about it, my dad and my sisters are probably depressed, too." This too may inflate estimates of familiality. Similarly, if assessors are not blinded to the proband diagnosis, they may be more apt to diagnose MDD in family members, introducing a similar bias.

In a meta-analysis, Sullivan and colleagues identified five studies using a family design which examined MDD [2]. All of them examined individuals with MDD drawn from clinic populations; one also included patients identified from the general population [3]. The comparator groups differed somewhat, ranging from individuals drawn from the general population and screened for MDD, to surgical patients not screened for psychiatric illness other than MDD. For the five studies, the overall odds ratio was 2.84 (95% CI 2.31–3.49) (that is, the ratio of the odds of depression among first-degree relatives of individuals with MDD, to odds of depression among first-degree relatives of individuals without MDD). Measures of effect were generally homogeneous across the individual studies, with ORs ranging from 2.21 to 4.57, with larger effects observed when the comparator subjects were screened to exclude psychiatric disorders other than MDD.

Is MDD risk inherited?

Early studies sought to determine inheritance patterns which might be informative about the genetic architecture of MDD. For example, some studies investigated whether MDD follows Mendelian (i.e. single-gene) inheritance patterns or more typically polygenic patterns [4]; and still others investigated the possibility of genetic anticipation (as is observed, for example, in disorders caused by trinucleotide repeat expansions such as Huntington's disease, where offspring tend to have earlier onset age than parents; see below). In general, patterns of inheritance are not suggestive of Mendelian or sex-linked inheritance, nor of genetic anticipation.

Twin studies

While family studies can establish the transmission of risk for MDD within a family, they cannot address whether this is genetic. This distinction, which may seem subtle at first, is actually critical. Families may share risk factors other than genes, particularly those related to environment – SES or degree of stress exposure, for example. Thus wealth tends to run in families (and indeed may be "inherited") but is hard to ascribe to genetics.

A sort of natural experiment which does allow the relative contribution of genes and environment to be addressed arises from twins. Comparing monozygotic twins, who share essentially 100% of DNA, and dizygotic twins, who like other sibling pairs share on average 50% of DNA, allows an estimate of the genetic contribution to disease risk. The most standard approach to studying twins models disease risk is in terms of three parameters: "shared" environmental effects (i.e. seen in both twins), "unique" environmental effects

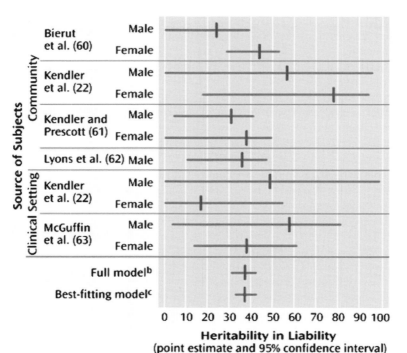

Figure 6.1 Estimates of the heritability in liability to major depression in studies of male and female twins, from P. F. Sullivan, M. C. Neale, and K. S. Kendler, Genetic epidemiology of major depression: review and meta-analysis, *Am J Psychiatry*, Oct 2000; 157: 1552–62. Reprinted with permission from the *American Journal of Psychiatry* (copyright 2000), American Psychiatric Association.

(i.e. those to which only one twin is exposed), and (additive) genetic effects. The mathematical models used to derive these parameters are addressed elsewhere [5].

The largest meta-analysis of twin studies [2] included four community-based (i.e. registry) cohorts and two clinical cohorts. Across the six studies, the overall estimate of genetic effects, or a^2, was 0.37 (95% CI 0.03–0.42). That is, 37% of the variance in risk for MDD was explained by genetic effects, with the remaining 63% of variance explained by individual environmental effects. (See Figure 6.1 adapted from [2], figure 1.) Importantly, despite subtle differences in methodologies and study populations, heritability estimates were generally consistent across studies. Moreover, the overall heritability appeared to be similar for males and females, despite the well-established difference in prevalence between genders [6].

Adoption studies

An alternative means of estimating genetic versus environmental effects is to examine the risk for MDD in adopted individuals. If environmental effects predominate, one would expect an individual's risk to be more similar to that of his or her adoptive parent. Conversely, if genetic effects predominate, one's risk should depend more strongly on the status of the biological parent.

Unfortunately, in contrast to the availability of large twin registries for study, adoption studies are somewhat less feasible and sometimes rely on very indirect phenotyping of biological parents. In the largest study to date [7], having a biological parent with MDD substantially increased one's risk for MDD – the estimated odds ratio was 7.2, although the confidence interval was wide (95% CI 1.2–43.2). In that study, subjects were not interviewed directly, which may limit the reliability of the assessments.

Another study [8] did not find increased risk of MDD in adopted offspring whose biological parents had MDD. However, that study examined male and female subgroups separately; a subsequent reanalysis [2] indicated that pooling the two subgroups does suggest elevated risk of MDD [OR 2.5, 95% CI 1.0–6.5].

Taken together, data from family, twin, and (to a lesser extent) adoption studies strongly suggest the heritability of MDD. From here, two broad categories of questions have been addressed. First, if genetic variation contributes to disease risk, can these individual genes be identified? Second, even in the absence of such findings, can patterns of inheritance be used to better characterize the nosology or etiology of MDD and related disorders? While the first question is in many ways the more straightforward, the second has arguably yielded more success so far. In the following sections, these are addressed in turn.

What genetic variations confer risk for MDD?

Long before it was feasible to investigate 500 000, 1 million, or more common genetic variations in a single experiment, it was possible to characterize a small number of variations spread across the 23 chromosomes. Because DNA is known to be inherited in "blocks," as a result of recombination, analysis of these patterns made it possible in some cases to determine whether an individual had inherited such a block from the mother or father. In its simplest form, one could then determine whether blocks "traveled with" disease risk. (For a more modern discussion of this block structure and its application in genetic investigation, see [9]). Particularly when extended pedigrees were available, allowing more precise estimates of how blocks of DNA were inherited, this approach could be extremely powerful, and indeed yielded great success in identifying many single-gene diseases.

The term applied to such studies is linkage analysis. Because of the relatively sparse coverage of the genome, these studies have been able to implicate regions of the genome as being more likely to harbor risk genes, but (as these regions may be many megabases in size and harbor many possible risk variants) cannot themselves implicate individual genetic variations.

Despite the large number of linkage studies conducted in MDD (or traits posited to contribute to MDD liability such as neuroticism; see discussion below), there is little consistency in which genomic regions are identified. Possible explanations for this discordance include sample heterogeneity (i.e. the studies are examining different phenotypes, or the regions differ by population), type I error (i.e. the linkage peaks are simply false positives), or type II error (i.e. because of limited power, many studies are simply unable to replicate findings from prior studies). Whatever the explanation, linkage studies in psychiatric disorders have not contributed to identification of disease genes thus far.

Genetic association studies

Initial investigations of genetic variation associated with MDD focused, by necessity, on a small number of variations which were more straightforward to assess. These studies are typically referred to as candidate gene studies – that is, genes (more properly variation in these genes) are identified as strong candidates for association with disease. Most often these are functional candidates – genes which, because of their function, would be expected to have a high prior probability of association with a disorder. Perhaps the best example of a functional candidate in MDD was the serotonin transporter (HTT, or SLC6A4), because it is the site of action of serotonin reuptake inhibitors such as fluoxetine, which are known to be effective treatments for MDD. Moreover, a vast literature underscores the importance of serotonin, and monoamines in general, in MDD (see chapters 1, 2 and 3). (The term functional is used in contrast to positional, as in a candidate gene is selected because it lies under a linkage peak.)

The design for genetic association studies as they pertain to MDD is typically rather simple. The frequency of a particular variation is examined in a group of (unrelated) affected individuals, who might be drawn from a psychiatric clinic or from the general population. This frequency is compared to that in a "control" group of individuals without MDD, ideally one which is otherwise very similar (in terms of ancestry) to the cases.

Summarizing the extensive literature on candidate gene studies in MDD would require a book unto itself. Instead, we highlight a few of the more consistent findings, and emphasize the limitations of this approach. The most intensively studied gene in psychiatry is undoubtedly the serotonin transporter (SLC6A4), responsible for uptake of serotonin from the synapse. As a proximal site of action of the most widely used class of antidepressants, the selective serotonin reuptake inhibitors (SSRIs), this gene has been considered among the strongest functional candidates for MDD. Moreover, a common variation in the promoter region of this gene in which a 44 base-pair region is present (inserted) or absent (deleted) was relatively straightforward to genotype and suggested to influence the degree to which this gene was transcribed, and thus the amount of transporter available.

In a seminal study, Caspi and colleagues found that the "short" variant was associated with increased risk of MDD, but only among individuals exposed to one or more "major life events" (i.e. stressors), and that the degree of risk was greater for individuals with multiple major life events [10]. This result, supported in some subsequent studies, had tremendous intellectual appeal because it seemed to nicely illustrate a model for gene-by-environment interactions: genes confer risk for MDD, but environment determines whether this liability becomes disease. Unfortunately, a later meta-analysis of 14 studies did not support this hypothesis, failing to confirm significant association between variation in the promoter region of SLC6A4 and depression liability (OR 1.05, 95% CI 0.98–1.13), or gene-by-environment interaction [11]. Thus, despite the appeal of the model, it does not appear to be supported by the bulk of recent evidence.

Most other candidate gene studies have examined the monoaminergic hypothesis of MDD, focusing on genes related to neurotransmitter metabolism, reuptake, or signaling, without consistent results. Another line of inquiry has considered the hypothesis that dysregulation in the hypothalamic–pituitary–adrenal (HPA) axis, and specifically the genes most important in HPA axis signaling, is associated with MDD risk. After an initial report of modest association between SNPs in the corticotropin-releasing hormone receptor-1 (CRHR1) gene and MDD [12], a subsequent report described an interaction between childhood abuse and CRHR1 SNPs in conferring MDD risk [13], and found similar effects in a second, smaller cohort. (Although it should also be noted that a large population-based study failed to find association between CRHR1 SNPs and MDD risk [14].)

An alternative to candidate-based studies which focus attention on one or a few genes is the genomewide association study (GWAS). For a full review of the GWAS approach and its application in psychiatry, see [15]. With this approach, it is possible to genotype at relatively modest cost 1 million or more variations "genome-wide." Taking advantage of the haplotype block structure of DNA – essentially, the correlation between nearby variations – it is also possible to "impute" additional SNPs in order to capture additional common genetic variation. In other words, in knowing which allele is carried at two other SNPs, it is often possible to impute the allele at the third SNP, even if it is not genotyped directly.

A key advantage of the GWAS approach compared to the candidate-based approach is the lack of bias towards well-characterized genes: in essence candidate gene studies can only confirm existing hypotheses, whereas GWAS may lead to truly novel findings. For example, outside of MDD, GWAS has frequently implicated genes and pathways which were not previously a focus of interest.

The breadth of coverage of GWAS also highlights its greatest disadvantage, namely that it is simultaneously testing ~1 MM hypotheses, and does not take into account any prior knowledge which might prioritize particular genes or pathways. As a result, the risk for type I error (so-called false positive results) is very high. The standard approach to control this type I error is to set a very high threshold for statistical significance, typically 5×10^{-8}. However, with this threshold, most association studies have very limited statistical power to detect all but the strongest associations. The most common solution to this problem is simply to increase sample size. Indeed, for other disorders such as bipolar disorder or schizophrenia, consistent results only began to emerge with sample sizes of ~3000–5000 or more (see, e.g., [16,17]).

In the first published study of MDD to use the GWAS approach, 1738 MDD cases and 1802 control subjects, no single SNP reached the threshold for declaring genome-wide significance [18]. However, multiple SNPs in a locus containing the synaptic gene piccolo (*PCLO*) were strongly suggestive of association (i.e. with *p*-values in the 10^{-6} to 10^{-7} range), so the authors and collaborators genotyped an additional 6079 cases and 5893 controls at multiple SNPs in *PCLO*, but failed to find evidence of replication in the combined cohorts. In post-hoc analyses, they suggested that heterogeneity among the individual cohorts may have contributed to non-replication, and indeed when the analysis was limited to the primary sample and the most similar follow-up sample, greater association was observed.

PCLO represents an intriguing functional candidate for further study in MDD because it is expressed in the presynaptic region and appears to play a role in monoaminergic neuro-transmission. Moreover, one of the SNPs with suggestive evidence of association in the GWAS is known to be a "coding" variation, as it changes the protein sequence, substituting an alanine for serine.

At least two other GWAS of MDD have been completed, with additional ones planned. While no single study has thus far found "genome-wide" evidence of association, it would be erroneous to conclude on this basis that such genes will not be identified. Indeed, for other psychiatric disorders such as bipolar disorder and schizophrenia, as well as complex diseases such as type II diabetes, consistent findings required sample sizes well in excess of those studied so far [16–19].

Beyond GWAS

Copy-number variation and other structural changes

While most genetic association studies in MDD focus on SNPs, another common type of interindividual variation is copy-number variation (CNV). This term describes changes in DNA including insertions, deletions, as well as multiple copies of a given region. Newer technologies for GWAS facilitate examination of CNV across the genome so its potential role in MDD, if any, may be characterized.

Larger-scale structural changes in DNA, such as translocations (in which a section of chromosome is shifted to another chromosome), can contribute to neurologic disorders with psychiatric features. In one well-characterized extended family in Scotland [20], a translocation on chromosome 1 [(1;11)(q42.1;q14.3)] has been associated with multiple psychiatric disorders ranging from schizophrenia to recurrent MDD. This translocation focused attention on the *DISC1* gene, disrupted by the translocation (thus its full name, Disrupted in Schizophrenia-1), as well as adjacent genes such as *TSNAX* (Translin-associated factor X) [21].

The role of trinucleotide repeats in MDD has also been investigated. Diseases associated with such repeats often exhibit anticipation, in which offspring are affected at a younger age than parents. This is not consistently the case in MDD, and where it is observed may arise from observer bias (that is, offspring of parents with MDD may simply be diagnosed at an earlier age because the parents' illness leads them to pursue evaluation for their children) [22]. However, depressive symptoms are commonly observed in individuals with heritable neuropsychiatric disorders including Parkinson's disease and Huntington's disease (HD), among many others, even before illness onset. One recent study found that 7 of ~3000 individuals diagnosed with MDD, and none of a similarly sized control group, exhibited expanded number of repeats in the Huntingtin gene which confers HD risk [23]. All but one of these were in a range which is incompletely penetrant for HD – that is, not all individuals with this number of repeats develop HD. Regardless of whether these individuals go on to develop the typical motor symptoms of HD, this finding suggests that some apparent cases of MDD may be associated with relatively rare genetic variation.

Common versus rare variation

To date, most identified disease genes for complex genetic diseases exhibit relatively modest effects. An elegant demonstration of the role of many genes of modest effect was provided by an analysis of GWAS data in schizophrenia [16]. In this report, rather than focusing on the top few associations, the authors examined whether including tens of thousands of associations (those with p-values less than 0.2 or even 0.5) improved their ability to identify disease risk for independent cohorts. That is, they compiled a "risk" score based on how many schizophrenia risk alleles were carried by a given individual. Remarkably, prediction ability improved even with the addition of these variants of very small effect. Using simulations, they suggested that about one-third of liability for schizophrenia might arise from common variation (that is, SNPs or other kinds of variation seen in at least 1% of the population).

On the other hand, some authors have criticized the "common gene" hypothesis, suggesting that identifying scores or hundreds of common variants, each of very small effect, will have little scientific or clinical utility [24]. They suggest instead that rare variants – for example, SNPs seen in only one or a few individuals, or rare CNVs – may contribute the majority of genetic risk. Such rare variants are more difficult to identify (typically requiring sequencing, or determining the base-by-base sequence of DNA) – at present, these studies focus on individual genes simply because of the cost and effort involved. One example of this approach identified novel variations in the brain-derived neurotrophic factor (BDNF) gene which were associated with MDD in a small cohort [25].

Epigenomics

An emerging area of interest in medical genetics is epigenetics and genomics. This concept refers to inherited factors other than DNA which may influence phenotype. (Importantly, it is also applied to changes which persist across cell divisions, even if not across generations – for example, where it plays a role in differentiation of tissue types.) While there are multiple potential types of epigenetic features, one which has received recent emphasis is the addition or removal of methyl groups at cytosine residues in DNA, typically in loci called CpG sites. (For a review of epigenetics in psychiatry, see [26]). This methylation may then influence the ability of proteins to bind to these sites, for example to initiate transcription of DNA into message RNA (mRNA).

Studies in MDD are beginning to emerge, but the role of tissue type in such studies remains unclear – for example, will studies in lymphocyte-derived cell lines yield similar results to those in brain tissue. As an example of the former, an analysis of methylation status in lymphoblastoid cell lines found numerically but not statistically greater levels of methylation in SLC6A4 among individuals with a history of MDD [27]. In the latter case, an analysis comparing brain tissue from suicide victims to control subjects who died of other causes revealed greater methylation in the promoter region of the GABA(A) receptor alpha1 subunit gene [28]. Notably, expression of this gene has been shown to be diminished in brains of individuals who die by suicide.

What is the right phenotype?

Major depressive disorder is so named in recognition that it likely does not represent a single disease, but rather a constellation of symptoms which may arise as a result of varied etiologies. There may be multiple "phenocopies" of MDD, phenotypes with a different genetic basis but overlapping phenotypes. If this is the case, many investigators have hypothesized that it might be possible to derive more specific phenotypes than MDD, which would facilitate the identification of causal genetic (or other inherited) variations.

One systematic means of identifying depressive subtypes for genetic study relies on family studies, asking which features of MDD render it most heritable. In other words, are there illness features seen more often in the relatives of individuals with MDD?

A typical study examined twin pairs to determine depressive features which might predict risk of MDD in the second twin [29]. Among 1765 twin-pairs in which at least one twin had a lifetime diagnosis of MDD, clinical features associated with MDD risk in the other twin included greater duration of longest mood episode, recurrent thoughts of death and suicide, and greater level of distress. Number of lifetime depressive episodes showed a complex relationship with risk to the co-twin, with risk increasing to a peak between seven and nine episodes and then decreasing again. Notably, while early age at onset has also been used to define a presumably more heritable phenotype, earlier age was not associated with greater risk to the co-twin in this cohort.

In general, little consistency has emerged across other investigations of familial aggregation, in part because they have rarely investigated overlapping illness features. A recent review indicated greatest consistency in association of impairment and recurrence [2], and lack of consistency for early onset of illness. Multiple different symptom patterns or subtypes have also shown suggestive evidence of familiality in individual studies.

An alternative means employed in the hope of identifying more genetically homogeneous subsets of MDD relies on the notion of endophenotypes or intermediate phenotypes. In essence, this approach posits that certain measurable traits might be more closely linked to the underlying pathophysiology of MDD, and thus more tightly associated to the genetic variations being sought. In the case of MDD, where the heritability is substantially less than (for example) bipolar disorder, finding a more heritable form might be expected to expedite the process of gene discovery. (For further discussion of endophenotypes, see [30].) Two major caveats must be considered here. First, within psychiatry, there are as yet no clear examples of endophenotypes successfully facilitating gene discovery. Even outside of psychiatry, in many cases putative endophenotypes were less helpful than the disorders themselves in finding associated variatiosn – see, for example, the case of type 2 diabetes. Second, even where an endophenotype is identified, there is no guarantee that it will be more heritable than MDD itself – the heritability of neuroimaging or neuropsychological phenotypes is generally not well characterized. (For an analogous discussion of endophenotypes in schizophrenia, see [31].)

Among the first endophenotypes to be considered were personality scales such as neuroticism or harm avoidance which have been linked to MDD risk, with the expectation that genes influencing temperament might also contribute to MDD. Neuroticism represents tendency to negative affective state [32], and has been associated with vulnerability to MDD in longitudinal studies [33,34]. Importantly, the heritability of neuroticism may be somewhat higher than that for MDD [35], which would support its use as an endophenotype. Multiple GWAS of neuroticism have been reported without clearly consistent results. For example, an analysis of 1227 healthy control subjects identified some SNPs with $p\sim10^{-6}$ which showed consistent association in a replication cohort of 1880 subjects [36], with the strongest association reported for a gene called *MAMDC1* (or *MDGA2*), suggested to regulate axonal guidance [37], although these did not reach the traditional threshold for genome-wide significance. Moreover, none of the most significant associations overlapped with those reported in a prior GWAS [38].

A host of other putative endophenotypes have been explored, with much recent emphasis placed on structural and functional neuroimaging. These approaches may be particularly useful in pursuing the functional implications of MDD risk genes "in vivo" as they are identified. While the association of SLC6A4 with MDD has been questioned, this model led to a line of intriguing functional MRI investigations demonstrating association between HTTLPR (the promoter insertion/deletion discussed earlier) and amygdala reactivity [39], a finding which has generally persisted in subsequent replication attempts [40]. In a similar vein, after an initial association was suggested between a variation in the *CREB1* gene and anger expression in MDD, functional MRI demonstrated that this variation appears to moderate activation of insula in healthy controls [41]. Traditionally when a genetic variation is associated with a disease, the bulk of follow-up involves in-vitro work – for example, demonstrating the effects of that variation on gene expression or regulation. However, these imaging studies suggest a parallel means by which association studies may be pursued.

Summary

Family studies indicate that MDD runs in families, although family members' risk for other psychiatric disorders may also be increased. Twin and adoption studies suggest that about one-third of the liability for MDD is inherited. However, to date, no single gene has been convincingly and consistently associated with MDD risk. As larger cohorts are examined using approaches which characterize variation across the genome, the likelihood of such consistent findings should increase. At the same time, investigations of other potential forms of inherited variation – rare genetic variation and epigenetic factors, for example – are ongoing. Results from other psychiatric disorders suggest that both common and rare genetic variation is likely to play a role in disease risk. Endophenotypes for MDD are also the subject of acute interest, although their value may be greater in characterizing rather than discovering causal variations.

References

1. Weissman M M, Merikangas K R, John K, Wickramaratne P, Prusoff B A, Kidd K K. Family genetic studies of psychiatric disorders. Developing technologies. *Arch Gen Psychiatry*. Nov 1986;**43**(11):1104–16.

2. Sullivan P F, Neale M C, Kendler K S. Genetic epidemiology of major depression: review and meta-analysis. *Am J Psychiatry*. Oct 2000;**157**(10):1552–62.

3. Weissman M M, Wickramaratne P, Adams P B, et al. The relationship between panic disorder and major depression. A new family study. *Arch Gen Psychiatry*. Oct 1993;**50**(10):767–80.

4. Smeraldi E, Negri F, Heimbuch R C, Kidd K K. Familial patterns and possible modes of inheritance of primary affective disorders. *J Affect Disord*. Jun 1981;**3**(2):173–82.

5. Neale M C, Cardon L R. *Methodology for the Study of Twins and Families*. Dordrecht, the Netherlands: Kluwer; 1992.

6. Kessler R C, Chiu W T, Demler O, Merikangas K R, Walters E E. Prevalence, severity, and comorbidity of 12-month DSM-IV disorders in the National Comorbidity Survey Replication. *Arch Gen Psychiatry*. Jun 2005;**62**(6):617–27.

7. Wender P H, Kety S S, Rosenthal D, Schulsinger F, Ortmann J, Lunde I. Psychiatric disorders in the biological and adoptive families of adopted individuals with affective disorders. *Arch Gen Psychiatry*. Oct 1986;**43**(10):923–29.

8. Cadoret R J, O'Gorman T W, Heywood E, Troughton E. Genetic and environmental factors in major depression. *J Affect Disord*. Sep 1985;**9**(2):155–64.

9. International HandMap Consortium. The International HapMap Project. *Nature*. Dec 18 2003;**426**(6968):789–96.

10. Caspi A, Sugden K, Moffitt T E, et al. Influence of life stress on depression: moderation by a polymorphism in the 5-HTT gene. *Science*. Jul 18 2003;**301**(5631):386–89.

11. Risch N, Herrell R, Lehner T, et al. Interaction between the serotonin transporter gene (5-HTTLPR), stressful life events, and risk of depression: a meta-analysis. *JAMA*. Jun 17 2009;**301**(23):2462–71.

12. Liu Z, Zhu F, Wang G, et al. Association of corticotropin-releasing hormone receptor1 gene SNP and haplotype with major depression. *Neurosci Lett*. Sep 1 2006;**404**(3):358–62.

13. Bradley R G, Binder E B, Epstein M P, et al. Influence of child abuse on adult depression: moderation by the corticotropin-releasing hormone receptor gene. *Arch Gen Psychiatry*. Feb 2008;**65**(2):190–200.

14. Utge S, Soronen P, Partonen T, et al. A population-based association study of candidate genes for depression and sleep disturbance. *Am J Med Genet B Neuropsychiatr Genet*. Jun 22 2009 [Epub ahead of print].

15. Cichon S, Craddock N, Daly M, et al. Genomewide association studies: history, rationale, and prospects for psychiatric disorders. *Am J Psychiatry*. May 2009;**166**(5):540–56.

16. Purcell S M, Wray N R, Stone J L, et al. Common polygenic variation contributes to risk of schizophrenia and bipolar disorder. *Nature* Aug 2009; **460**(7256):748–52.

17. Ferreira M A, O'Donovan M C, Meng Y A, et al. Collaborative genome-wide association analysis supports a role for ANK3 and CACNA1C in bipolar disorder. *Nat Genet*. Sep 2008;**40**(9):1056–58.

18. Sullivan P F, de Geus E J, Willemsen G, et al. Genome-wide association for major depressive disorder: a possible role for the presynaptic protein piccolo. *Mol Psychiatry*. Apr 2009;**14**(4):359–75.

19. Zeggini E, Scott L J, Saxena R, et al. Meta-analysis of genome-wide association data and large-scale replication identifies additional susceptibility loci for type 2 diabetes. *Nat Genet*. May 2008;**40**(5):638–45.

20. St Clair D, Blackwood D, Muir W, et al. Association within a family of a balanced autosomal translocation with major mental illness. *Lancet*. Jul 7 1990;**336**(8706):13–16.

21. Schosser A, Gaysina D, Cohen-Woods S, et al. Association of DISC1 and TSNAX genes and affective disorders in the depression case-control (DeCC) and bipolar affective case-control (BACCS) studies. *Mol Psychiatry*. Mar 3 2009 [Epub ahead of print].

22. Papadimitriou G N, Souery D, Lipp O, et al. In search of anticipation in unipolar affective disorder. *Eur Neuropsychopharmacol*. Oct 2005;**15**(5):511–16.

23. Perlis R H, Smoller J W, Mysore J, et al. Prevalence of incompletely penetrant Huntington's Disease alleles among individuals with major depressive disorder. *Am J Psychiatry*, in press.

24. Goldstein D B. Common genetic variation and human traits. *N Engl J Med*. Apr 23 2009;**360**(17):1696–98.

25. Licinio J, Dong C, Wong M L. Novel sequence variations in the brain-derived neurotrophic factor gene and association with major depression and antidepressant treatment response. *Arch Gen Psychiatry*. May 2009;**66**(5):488–97.

26. Tsankova N, Renthal W, Kumar A, Nestler E J. Epigenetic regulation in psychiatric disorders. *Nat Rev Neurosci*. May 2007;**8**(5):355–67.

27. Philibert R A, Sandhu H, Hollenbeck N, Gunter T, Adams W, Madan A. The relationship of 5HTT (SLC6A4) methylation and genotype on mRNA expression and liability to major depression and alcohol dependence in subjects from the Iowa Adoption Studies. *Am J Med Genet B Neuropsychiatr Genet*. Jul 5 2008;**147B**(5):543–49.

28. Poulter M O, Du L, Weaver I C, et al. GABAA receptor promoter hypermethylation in suicide brain: implications for the involvement of epigenetic processes. *Biol Psychiatry*. Oct 15 2008;**64**(8):645–52.

29. Kendler K S, Gardner C O, Prescott C A. Clinical characteristics of major depression that predict risk of depression in relatives. *Arch Gen Psychiatry*. Apr 1999;**56**(4):322–27.

30. Gottesman, I I, Gould T D. The endophenotype concept in psychiatry: etymology and strategic intentions. *Am J Psychiatry*. Apr 2003;**160**(4):636–45.

31. Greenwood T A, Braff D L, Light G A, et al. Initial heritability analyses of endophenotypic measures for schizophrenia: the consortium on the genetics of schizophrenia. *Arch Gen Psychiatry*. Nov 2007;**64**(11):1242–50.

32. Costa P T, Jr., McCrae R R. Influence of extraversion and neuroticism on subjective well-being: happy and unhappy people. *J Pers Soc Psychol*. Apr 1980;**38**(4):668–78.

33. Ormel J, Oldehinkel A J, Vollebergh W. Vulnerability before, during, and after a major depressive episode: a 3-wave population-based study. *Arch Gen Psychiatry*. Oct 2004;**61**(10):990–96.

34. Kendler K S, Gatz M, Gardner C O, Pedersen N L. Personality and major depression: a Swedish longitudinal, population-based twin study. *Arch Gen Psychiatry*. Oct 2006;**63**(10):1113–20.

35. Lake R I, Eaves L J, Maes H H, Heath A C, Martin N G. Further evidence against the environmental transmission of individual differences in neuroticism from a collaborative study of 45,850 twins and relatives on two continents. *Behav Genet*. May 2000;**30**(3):223–33.

36. van den Oord E J, Kuo P H, Hartmann A M, et al. Genomewide association analysis followed by a replication study implicates a novel candidate gene for neuroticism. *Arch Gen Psychiatry*. Sep 2008;**65**(9):1062–71.

37. Litwack E D, Babey R, Buser R, Gesemann M, O'Leary D D. Identification and characterization of two novel brain-derived immunoglobulin superfamily members with a unique structural organization. *Mol Cell Neurosci*. Feb 2004;**25**(2):263–74.

38. Shifman S, Bhomra A, Smiley S, et al. A whole genome association study of neuroticism using DNA pooling. *Mol Psychiatry*. Mar 2008;**13**(3):302–12.

39. Hariri A R, Mattay V S, Tessitore A, et al. Serotonin transporter genetic variation and the response of the human amygdala. *Science*. Jul 19 2002;**297** (5580):400–03.

40. Munafo M R, Brown S M, Hariri A R. Serotonin transporter (5-HTTLPR) genotype and amygdala activation: a meta-analysis. *Biol Psychiatry*. May 1 2008;**63**(9):852–57.

41. Perlis R H, Holt D J, Smoller J W, et al. Association of a polymorphism near CREB1 with differential aversion processing in the insula of healthy participants. *Arch Gen Psychiatry*. Aug 2008;**65**(8):882–92.

Medicinal chemistry challenges in the design of next generation antidepressants

David P. Rotella

Abstract

Monoamine-based strategies and targets have provided a useful variety of therapeutic agents with beneficial activity in the treatment of depression. However, this approach has some limitations, including a delayed onset of efficacy and treatment resistance. As a result, there is significant interest in non-monoamine targets and their potential as antidepressants. This search for new treatment modalities has been aided by better understanding of the neurochemical pathways involved in mood. This chapter will review medicinal chemistry advances in a selection of non-monoamine targets of current interest in the field.

Introduction

The efficacy of tricyclic antidepressants such as imipramine, **1**, and amitriptyline, **2** (Figure 7.1) for treatment of depression in the 1950s marked the beginning of a chemotherapeutic approach for this widespread disorder [1]. These compounds and their desmethyl metabolites nortriptyline, **3** and desipramine, **4** were subsequently discovered to exert their activity on a variety of neurotransmitter systems in the central nervous systems. In particular, these compounds were found to inhibit reuptake of norepinephrine and serotonin and antagonize histamine receptors.

Better understanding of the neurochemistry associated with depression led to a focus on the neurotransmitter serotonin, because of the implied association with mood [2]. It was well known that administration of reserpine, which depletes serotonin, can lead to clinical depression [3]. The hypothesis that elevation of serotonin concentration in the brain would improve mood was tested by serotonin reuptake inhibitors, typified by fluoxetine, **5**, and followed by sertraline, **6**, paroxetine, **7**, citalopram, **8**, and fluvoxamine, **9** (Figure 7.2). The clinical success of these agents, and their improved tolerability and safety profile, compared to first generation agents such as imipramine, validated the serotonergic hypothesis and established this class of compounds as important therapeutic options [4].

A substantial body of clinical experience has shown that these selective serotonin reuptake inhibitors (SSRIs), while effective in many patients, have drawbacks. Among these, delayed onset of efficacy and treatment resistance are noteworthy. Three to six weeks of SSRI administration are typically required before significant antidepressant effects are

Next Generation Antidepressants: Moving Beyond Monoamines to Discover Novel Treatment Strategies for Mood Disorders, ed. Chad E. Beyer and Stephen M. Stahl. Published by Cambridge University Press.
© Cambridge University Press 2010.

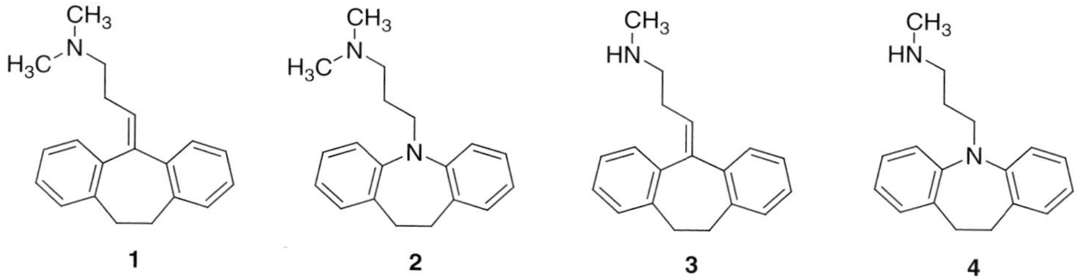

Figure 7.1 Structure of 1–4.

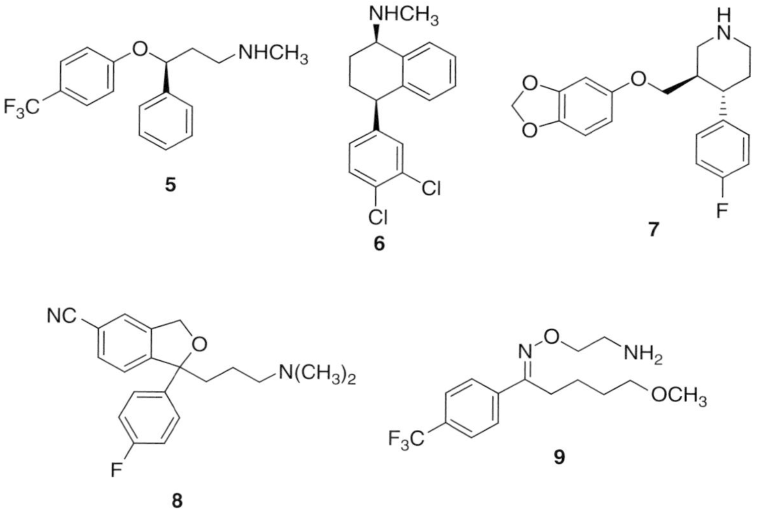

Figure 7.2 Structure of 5–9.

observed in humans. This delay has been attributed to a variety of factors, including $5HT_{1A}$ receptor desensitization, stimulation of neurogenesis, alterations of synaptic signaling and intracellular signal transduction and gene expression [5–10]. It has been estimated that up to 30% of patients, when treated with maximally tolerated doses for an appropriate period of time, do not respond to approved chemotherapeutic options [11]. These observations have been cited as evidence in favor of the hypothesis that elevation of synaptic neurotransmitters is the initial step in a process that also should involve the biochemical and structural changes outlined above [12,13].

Dual serotonin/norepinephrine reuptake inhibitors (SNRIs) such as venlafaxine, **10**, its active metabolite desvenlafaxine **11**, duloxetine, **12**, and milnacipran, **13** (Figure 7.3) may have advantages over SSRIs in terms of a somewhat more rapid onset of action, and possibly improved efficacy [14]. A retrospective comparison of fluoxetine and venlafaxine indicated that the SNRI demonstrated greater efficacy compared to the SSRI [15]. In spite of this potential, SNRIs are not always the treatment of choice in all patients because of pre-existing comorbidities such as hypertension [16]. Additionally, treatment resistance has been reported in patients treated with SNRIs, tolerability remains an issue, and the onset of action is not immediate. This last feature is a major contributing factor to treatment efficacy for both SSRIs and SNRIs [14].

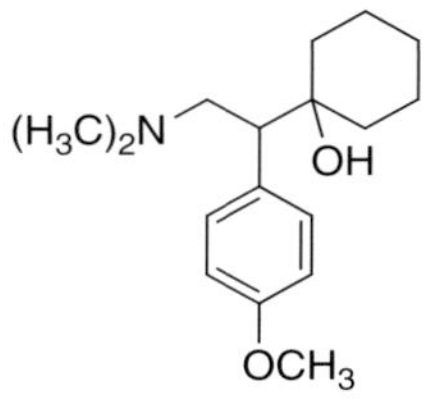

Figure 7.3 Structure of **10–13**.

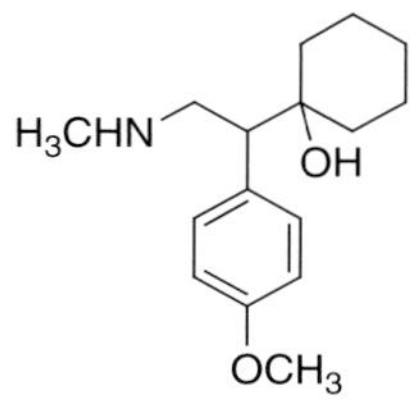

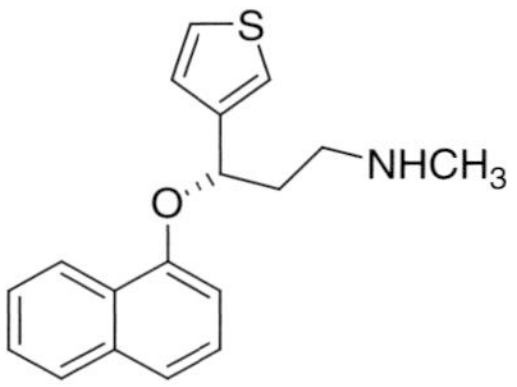

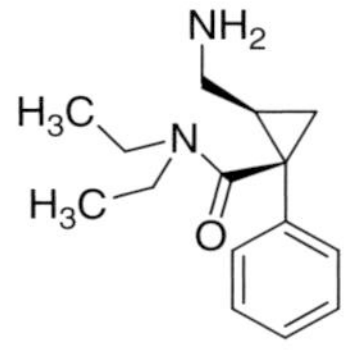

Improved understanding of disease pathophysiology, genetics, environmental factors, and the range of neurochemical pathways that are affected by and influence mood will all contribute to the development of agents that address these unmet needs. The development of animal models that allow researchers to evaluate these contributing factors will also play an important role in the discovery of new antidepressant therapies. This chapter will survey selected potential multitarget approaches and non-monoamine-based therapeutic targets that are of current interest in the field.

Potential multitarget approaches

As noted above and elsewhere in this volume, there are a variety of neurotransmitter systems that can influence mood, including monoaminergic systems for serotonin, norepinephrine, and dopamine, as well as glutaminergic receptors. Given the significant number of patients who do not respond to, or cannot tolerate, an antidepressant primarily designed to target a single neurotransmitter, the possibility of specifically designing novel molecules that exert activity at more than one receptor is a concept that has been, and continues to be, an approach for the discovery of potential antidepressants.

Selective serotonin reuptake inhibitors combined with 5HT$_{1A}$ receptor antagonism

One hypothesis that can explain the delayed onset of action of SSRIs invokes the time required to desensitize presynaptic 5HT$_{1A}$ autoreceptors by elevated levels of serotonin [17]. A combination of serotonin reuptake inhibition with 5HT$_{1A}$ receptor antagonism may shorten the time required for onset of antidepressant activity. Administration of WAY-100635, a selective 5HT$_{1A}$ antagonist, prior to dosing with the SSRIs citalopram, fluoxetine, and fluvoxamine, resulted in immediate increases in serotonin levels in the frontal cortex of rats, as measured by microdialysis [18]. This neurochemical observation was supported by animal studies where WAY-100635 was administered in combination with paroxetine to rats. This led to a shortened time for a positive response in a social interaction model [19].

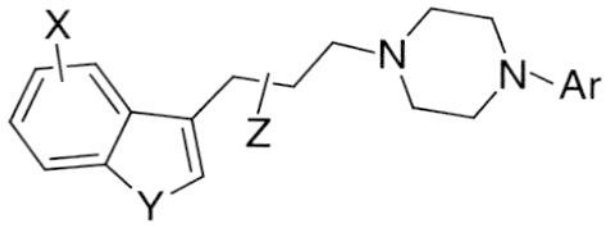

Figure 7.4 Example of an SSRI-5HT$_{1A}$ pharmacophore. X = H, F, CN, Cl; Y = NH, S; Z = alkyl, alkoxy.

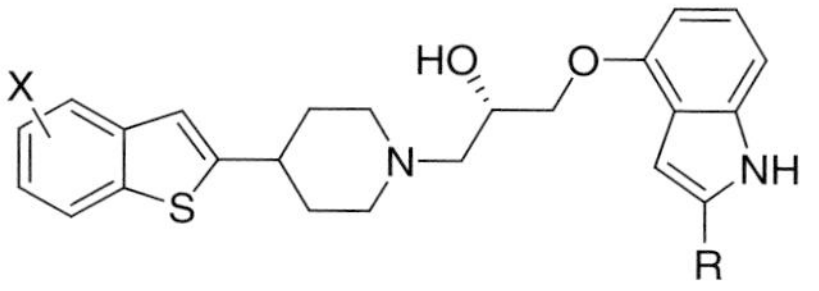

14 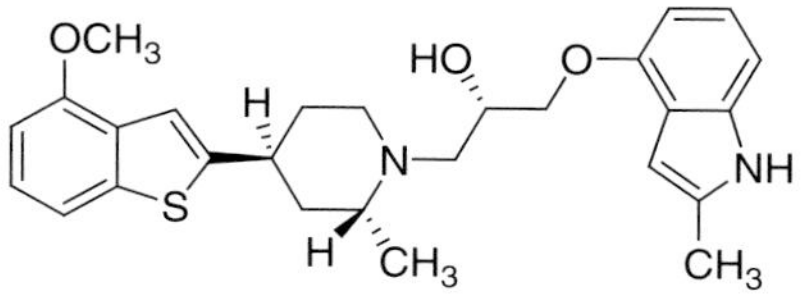   15

Figure 7.5 Structure of **14** and **15**.

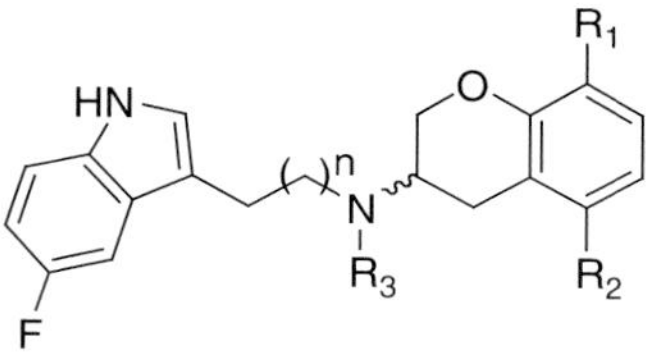

16 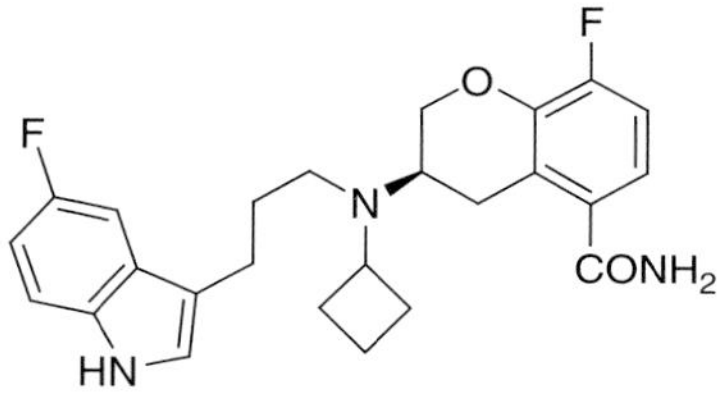   17

Figure 7.6 Structure of **16** and **17**.

The discovery of dual SSRI-5HT$_{1A}$ antagonists has been investigated by a number of groups. The general medicinal chemistry strategy has been to combine the respective pharmacophores, e.g. a 3-propylamino substituted indole or benzothiophene as the SSRI component, and an aryl piperazine 5HT$_{1A}$ fragment, into a single molecule using the basic secondary nitrogen atom, that both fragments share. One example of this is shown in Figure 7.4.

One well-investigated series of compounds employed the 5HT$_{1A}$ antagonist pindolol and its derivatives with piperidinyl benzothiophene-based SSRI building blocks, as in **14** (Figure 7.5) [20]. It was found that electron-donating substituents on the benzothiophene reduced SSRI activity without a large effect on 5HT$_{1A}$ antagonism, and electron-withdrawing groups, especially a 6-fluoro analog, generally were more potent at the SSRI site, and maintained 5HT$_{1A}$ activity below 10 nM as antagonists. In subsequent developments, this template was modified, leading to a series of compounds exemplified by **15** [21], that demonstrated in-vivo activity at both receptor targets and in microdialysis studies in rats showed a substantial increase in serotonin in the hypothalamus, compared to a combination of fluoxetine and WAY-100635.

A different set of SSRI and 5HT$_{1A}$ building blocks were employed by Hatzenbuhler et al. as a part of their efforts to identify dual-acting compounds [22]. Using a chroman as the 5HT$_{1A}$ component and 3-alkylamino indoles as the SSRI portion (**16**, Figure 7.6), this SAR study evaluated the length of the alkyl linker, substituents on the secondary amine and on the chroman. It was found that 5HT$_{1A}$ activity was dependent on the basic nitrogen substituent, and preferred compounds contained either cyclobutyl or methylcyclopropyl

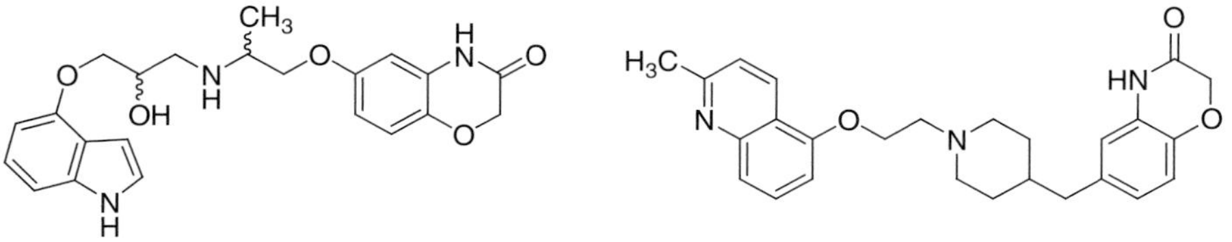

Figure 7.7 Structure of **18** and **19**.

groups. The absolute stereochemistry at the chroman also played an important role as a determinant of $5HT_{1A}$ activity, where compounds with R-absolute stereochemistry more consistently showed antagonism. Chain length played a role in determining serotonin reuptake inhibition, and optimal activity was obtained with a 3- or 4-carbon chain. One compound in this series, **17**, showed greater than 100-fold selectivity versus other mono-amine receptors, and demonstrated the ability to acutely (within 30 min) elevate serotonin in the frontal cortex of rats following an oral dose of 30 mg/kg. The acute microdialysis response to compound **17** was comparable to that observed following chronic (14 day) administration of an SSRI, demonstrating its possible immediate onset activity in raising serotonin levels [23,24].

In another approach to SSRI/$5HT_{1A}$ antagonists, a combination of benzoxazinones, as the SSRI pharmacophore, and quinolines, as the $5HT_{1A}$ fragment, provide dual-acting compounds, some of which showed oral bioavailability and brain penetration [25]. High-throughput screening identified a benzoxazinone derivative (**18**, Figure 7.7) as a lead structure. This lead was modified in the linker region and by replacing the pindolol-like $5HT_{1A}$ antagonist portion with other $5HT_{1A}$ pharmacophores. It was found that a piper-idine ring attached to the benzoxazinone by a methylene unit, and a 2-methyl quinoline $5HT_{1A}$ antagonist unit provided a compound, SB-649915 (**19**), with acute activity in rodent models of depression [26,27]. When tested in acute models of depression, such as rat pup vocalization and marmoset human threat, **19** showed an ED_{50} of 0.17 mg/kg ip in the former, and significant activity at 3 and 10 mg/kg when administered subcutaneously in the latter. In a rat high light social interaction chronic model, oral administration of SB-649915 three times daily 1 and 3 mg/kg doses increased social interaction time without an affect on locomotion at day 7. The SSRI paroxetine did not show activity in this model until day 21.

Triple reuptake inhibitors

As noted previously, inhibition of serotonin and norepinephrine reuptake activity in a single molecule has provided clinically effective antidepressant agents. Extension of this concept to include dopamine, a third monoamine neurotransmitter associated with mood, has advanced to clinical evaluation for efficacy using DOV 21947 (**20**, Figure 7.8), a compound currently in phase II trials. DOV 21947 has K_i values of 66, 262, and 213 nM, for the serotonin, norepinephrine, and dopamine reuptake sites, respectively [28]. The rationale for combining all three activities into a single molecule is based on a range of preclinical and clinical observations that couple dopaminergic function to anhedonia, a well-known symptom in patients with anxiety and depression [29,30]. It has been

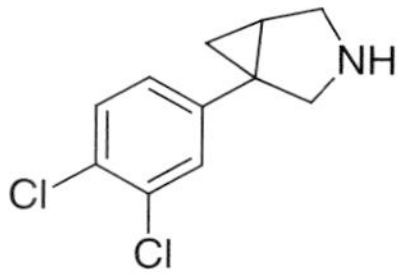

Figure 7.8 Structure of **20–22**.

hypothesized that a triple reuptake inhibitor may distinguish itself from SSRIs and SNRIs by exerting antidepressant activity more rapidly [31]. A second potential advantage associated with triple reuptake inhibitors may be reduced incidence of sexual dysfunction seen with SSRIs due to the role dopamine plays in the release of prolactin [32]. The lack of sexual side effects has been demonstrated with the racemic isomer of **20**, DOV 216,303 at doses that were active in a chronic rat olfactory bulbectomy model [33].

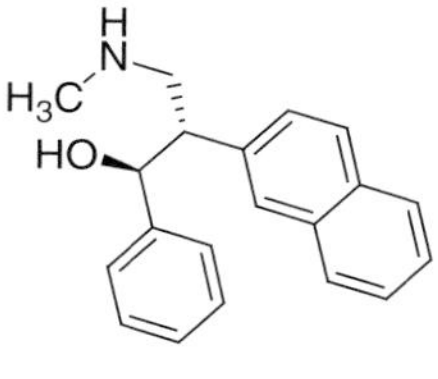

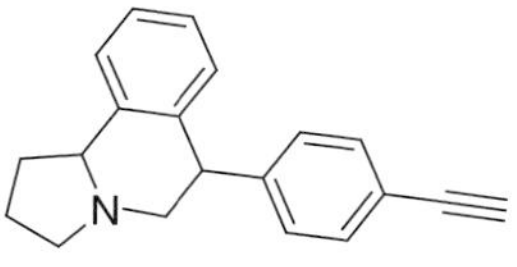

A structurally distinct triple reuptake inhibitor, PRC200-SS (**21**, Figure 7.8) was developed by systematic modification of the venlafaxine template [34,35]. This particular diastereomer is the most active of the other isomers of the racemic analog, and has K_i values of 2.1, 1.5, and 61 nM, for serotonin, norepinephrine, and dopamine reuptake inhibition, respectively. Using a rat forced swim model, **21** dose-dependently decreased immobility and increased mobility. In this assay, PRC200-SS, at a dose of 1 mg/kg, showed activity comparable to a 15 mg/kg dose of imipramine. Comparable effects were observed at 5 and 10 mg/kg of **21**. In a mouse tail suspension test, at 0.5 mg/kg, **21** demonstrated activity comparable to imipramine at 15 mg/kg. No significant locomotor effects were noted in mice at the active doses, while a 5 mg/kg dose in rats stimulated locomotor activity, but no effect was observed at 1 or 10 mg/kg. Unlike cocaine, which induces self-administration, **21** did not induce self-administration at a 1 mg/kg infusion rate over 7 days in rats.

JNJ-7925476, **22** (Figure 7.8), is another recent example of a structurally distinct triple reuptake inhibitor that demonstrates antidepressant activity in the mouse tail suspension assay, with an ED_{50} of 0.3 mg/kg ip. The racemate has K_i values of 0.9, 17, and 5.2 nM, respectively, for 5-HT, NE, and DA uptake inhibition. In rat brain, the compound shows ED_{50} values for receptor occupancy of 0.18, 0.09, and 2.4 mg/kg, respectively, and rapidly induced dose-dependent increases in extracellular levels of these neurotransmitters in cerebral cortex [36].

Using perceived key structural features in DOV 216303 (**20**) and a known indolyl phenylpropylamino series (**23**) of SNRIs, triple reuptake inhibitors were designed by Bannwart et al. (Figure 7.9) [37]. This work focused on structure-activity development of a 3,3-disubstituted pyrrolidine template. Using a 3-benzyl pyrrolidine core, 3-, 5-, and 6-indoles, along with heterocyclic indazole, 7-azaindole, and benzothiophenyl analogs were prepared to investigate the SAR of the pendant aryl (or heteroaryl) moiety. Many of these derivatives demonstrated potent NE-reuptake inhibition, with K_i values less than 5 nM. A wider range of activity was observed at the dopamine reuptake channel, where K_i values varied from 11 nM to greater than 1 micromolar. Serotonin reuptake inhibition in all compounds showed K_i values less than 200 nM, with some compounds below 10 nM.

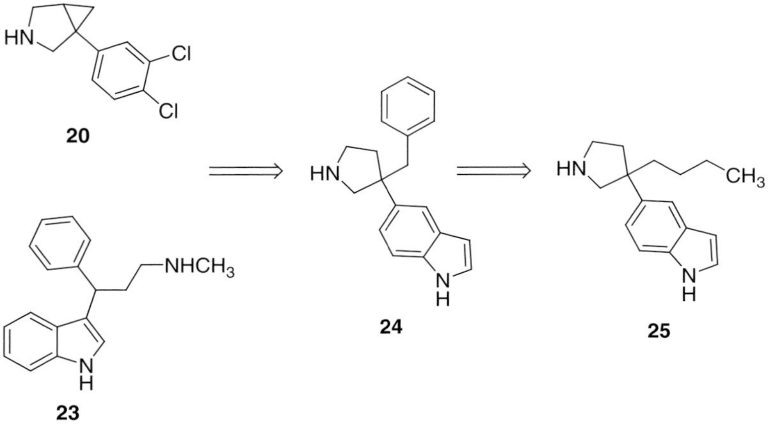

Figure 7.9 Structure of **20** and **23–25**.

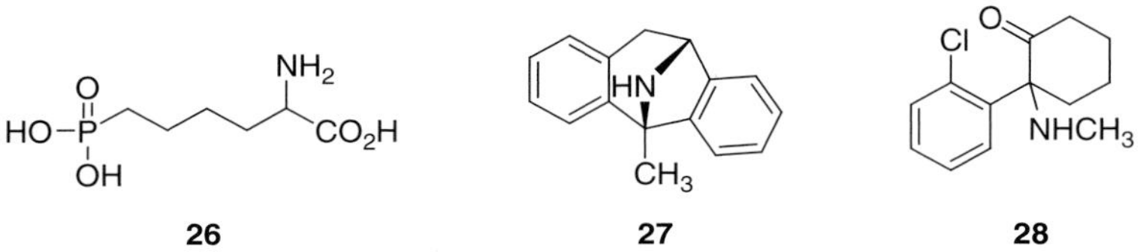

20

23

24

25

Figure 7.10 Structure of **26–28**.

26

27

28

Benzyl derivatives at the 3-position on the pyrrolidine showed potent triple reuptake activity, but this was accompanied by CYP inhibition, hERG affinity, and low in-vitro microsomal stability. These properties were attenuated by replacement of the benzyl group with short alkyl chains. *n*-Propyl and *n*-butyl derivatives, e.g. **24**, represented the best balance between triple reuptake inhibition potency and pharmaceutical properties in this set of analogs. One derivative, indolyl analog **25**, was active following ip administration at 30 mg/kg in a mouse tail suspension assay.

Glutamatergic targets

Glutaminergic signaling plays a key role in mood disorders, and is a regulator of neuro-chemical pathways associated with mood. NMDA antagonists AP-7, **26**, and MK-801 (**27**, Figure 7.10) showed activity in animal models of depression, such as forced swim, tail suspension, and open field activity [38]. This was followed by neurochemically focused studies that revealed the association between glutamate receptor expression and function and chronic antidepressant therapies [39–41]. The NMDA antagonist ketamine, **28**, rapidly expresses antidepressant activity in humans that persists even after drug administration ceases, and is efficacious in a high percentage of treatment-resistant patients [42].

Among the various potential glutamatergic receptor targets, e.g. NR2B, NMDA, and the mGluR family, the mGluR5 receptor has received a significant amount of attention in recent years. The prototypical mGluR5 antagonists, MPEP, **29**, and the more selective MTEP, **30** (Figure 7.11), have been widely used as standards in a variety of in-vivo and neurochemical studies to characterize the role this receptor plays in mood control [43–45]. A number of approaches to the modulation of this receptor have been investigated, including direct and allosteric mGluR5 receptor modulation, and a range of chemotypes

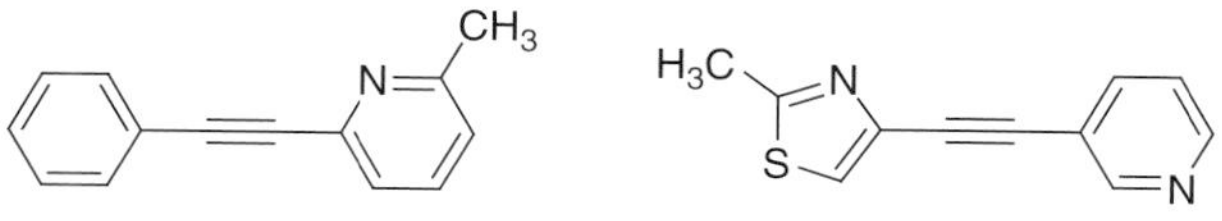

Figure 7.11 Structure of **29** and **30**.

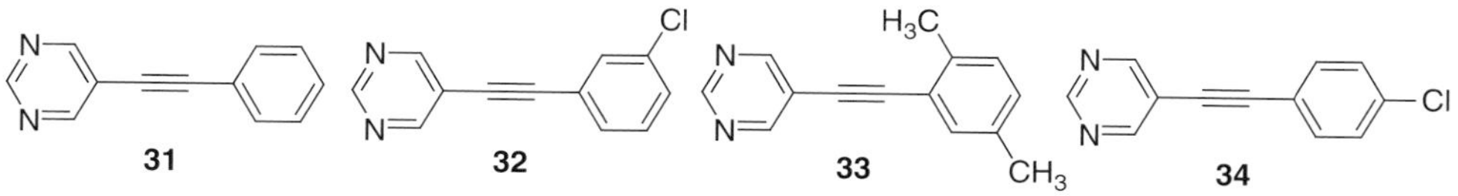

Figure 7.12 Structure of **31–34**.

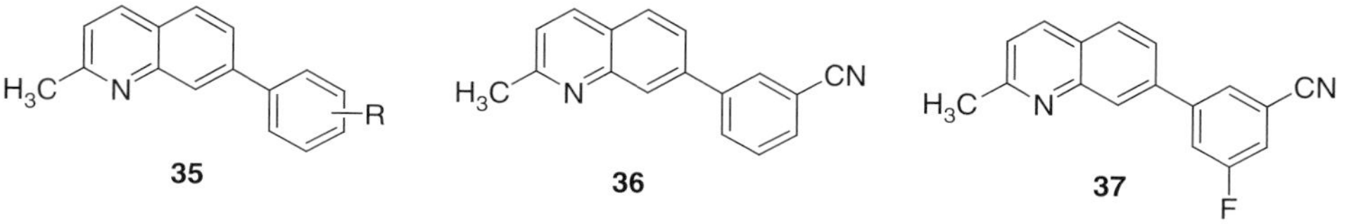

Figure 7.13 Structure of **35–37**.

active at this receptor have been reported. Selected examples of mGluR5-active compounds are highlighted below, including, where possible, specific mention of compounds that have demonstrated activity in preclinical models of depression.

The functional activity of mGluR5 ligands related to MPEP was recently reported by Sharma and co-workers [46]. MPEP and MTEP are non-competitive antagonists that bind to an allosteric site on the receptor, and they function as inverse agonists to block constitutive activity [47]. The complete cessation of receptor signaling may result in cognitive deficits or undesired psychotomimetic activity [48]. Previous studies identified compounds that functioned as partial antagonists [48], and based on this work, a high throughput screen identified an alkynylpyrimidine lead, **31** (Figure 7.12), that was shown to displace an MPEP derivative with a K_i value of 125 nM. Substitutions on the phenyl ring with electron-donating and -withdrawing groups provided analogs with a range of affinity (7–18 800 nM), and a range of functional activities, from complete antagonists, e.g. **32**, to partial antagonists, e.g. **33**, to positive allosteric modulators, e.g. **34**. SAR analysis indicated that substituents attached at the 3-position resulted in full antagonists, while 4-substitution provided positive allosteric modulators that provide nearly complete functional responses when stimulated by glutamate.

It has been shown that the presence of an acetylene functional group in potentially biologically active molecules can elicit properties associated with activation of CYP enzymes and catalyzed or uncatalyzed addition of glutathione, which may lead to idiosyncratic or hepatic toxicity [49]. In an effort to identify mGluR5 antagonists structurally distinct from acetylene-based compounds such as MTEP or those in Figure 7.12, an aromatic ring can be installed on the diaryl acetylene template to take the place of the triple bond. This approach was investigated by Milbank and co-workers, within the context of a 7-arylquinoline core structure **35** (Figure 7.13) [49]. In this series, monosubstitution on the pendant aryl ring furnished compounds with much lower affinity (>400 nM)

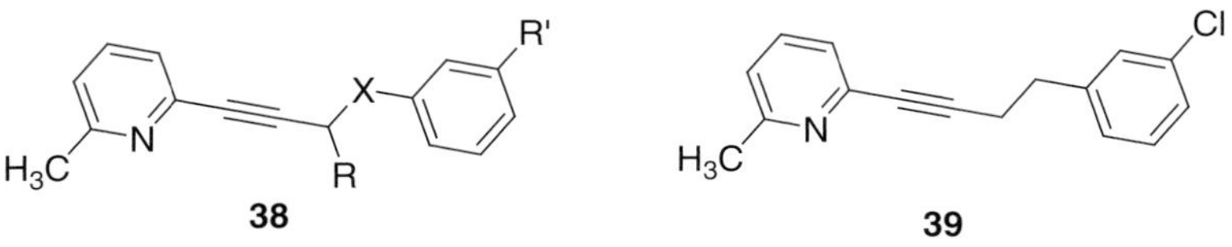

Figure 7.14
Structure of **38**
and **39**.

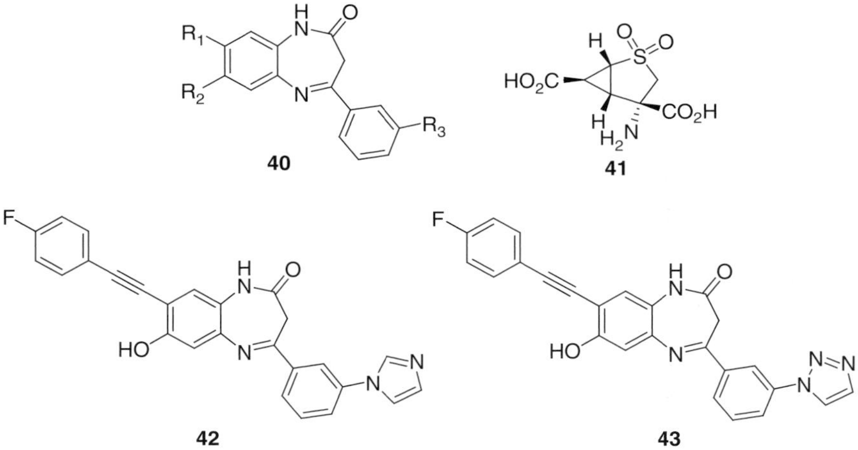

Figure 7.15 Structure of **40–43**.

compared to MPEP, with the exception of a 3-cyano analog, **36**, with an IC_{50} value of 7.7 nM (MPEP IC_{50} 0.2 nM). Addition of a second substituent to the phenyl ring at the 5-position provided compounds with a wide range of activity (FLIPR IC_{50}s 0.8–12 000 nM), with the 5-F analog **37** as the most potent derivative. This compound was tested in the Vogel assay for anti-anxiety activity and showed 100% reversal of punished drinking behavior compared to control after an oral dose of 10 mg/kg. In this assay, MPEP showed comparable efficacy at the same dose.

Bach et al. reported linker modifications in a group of pyridinyl alkynes, **38** [50]. In, addition to inserting various heteroatoms, this group also evaluated carbonyl- and heterocycle-based derivatives. Direct comparison of mGluR5 binding for these new compounds with MPEP or MTEP was not reported. The most active derivative was a two-carbon linker containing a 3-chlorophenyl moiety, **39** (Figure 7.14), with an mGluR5 binding IC_{50} of 5 nM. This compound showed no binding activity at mGluR1 receptors. Heteroatom, carbonyl derivatives (amides, ureas) and heterocycle derivatives (benzothiophenes) were less active. Compound **39** was tested in a gastroesophageal efflux model by iv administration, and at a dose of 3.9 μmol/kg, inhibited lower esophageal sphincter relaxation by 31%. At a dose of 8.7 μmol/kg iv, MPEP inhibited sphincter relaxation by 59%.

mGluR2/3 receptors have also attracted recent attention in the search for novel antidepressant agents. In the brain, these receptors have been localized in regions of the cortex and dentate gyrus, and have been found both presynaptically and postsynaptically [51–54] and activity of antagonists in preclinical animal models of depression has been established [55,56]. Two reports from Woltering and co-workers described the optimization of a series of benzodiazepine derivatives, **40** (Figure 7.15), as non-competitive

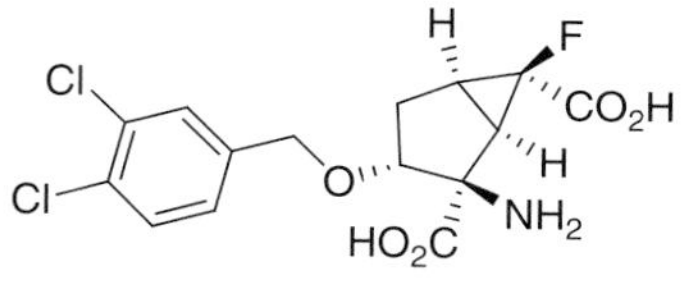

Figure 7.16
Structure of **44** and **45**.

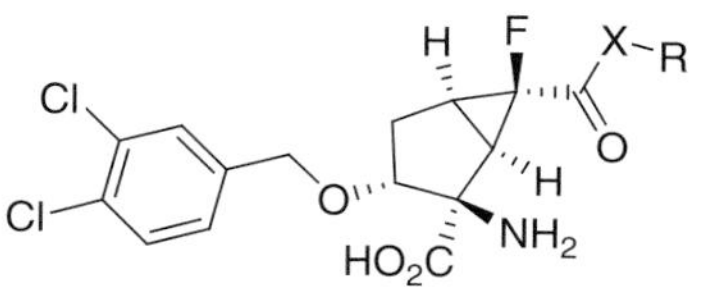

mGluR2/3 antagonists [57,58]. Installation of a phenyl-propynyl moiety at R2 resulted in improved affinity, and an alkoxyl-linked polar moiety at R1 led to further enhancement in activity [57]. More detailed SAR exploration identified two compounds with good potency and functional activity as mGluR2/3 antagonists, **42** (IC$_{50}$ 26 nM) and **43** (IC$_{50}$ 20 nM). These molecules showed the ability to reverse the binding of an mGluR2/3 agonist, LY354740 (**41**), in the dentate gyrus [58].

MGS0039, **44** (Figure 7.16), is a potent, selective mGluR2/3 antagonist that is structurally related to LY354740 [59]. In an attempt to improve the oral bioavailability of this derivative, a series of prodrugs were reported by Yasuhara and co-workers [60]. Dipeptide derivatives attached via the cyclopropane carboxyl moiety (**45** X = NH, R = various dipeptides) were not cleaved in rat liver microsomal preparations. However, a variety of alkyl esters at the same position (**45**, X = O, R = branched and straight chain alkyl, cycloalkyl) were cleaved to **44** in microsomal preparations, and following oral administration to rats, improved bioavailability was noted (up to 66%). A heptyl ester prodrug of **44** was tested in rats in a forced swim model. A dose-dependent effect was observed, with a minimally efficacious dose at 3 mg/kg orally. A similar dose response effect was seen in a tail suspension assay in mice. At 3 and 10 mg/kg oral doses, the heptyl ester prodrug did not influence spontaneous locomotor activity in rats or mice. However, in rats only, locomotor activity increased at 30 mg/kg. Analysis of plasma in test animals showed low levels of prodrug at key timepoints associated with the antidepressant assays.

Orphanin FQ/nociceptin receptor agonists

The orphanin FQ/nociceptin receptor was discovered by analysis of a human cDNA library and was identified as a member of the opioid receptor family. Compounds with agonist and antagonist activity, and with selective activity against the NOP-1/ORL-1 receptor have been identified [61]. The NOP-1 receptor was shown to be a potential target for antidepressant drug therapy when Ro64–6198, **46** (Figure 7.17), demonstrated activity in preclinical studies [62]. More recently, the detailed pharmacological characterization of two structurally distinct NOP-1 agonists have been reported.

Compound **47**, SCH 221510 [63], a potent (K$_i$ 0.3 nM), full (EC$_{50}$ 12 nM) NOP-1 agonist, with at least 200-fold selectivity for other opioid receptors was tested in a variety of antidepressasnt assays in rats and mice. In a rat elevated plus maze model, orally administered **47** significantly increased the time spent in the open arms at a dose of 1 mg/kg, and dose-dependently increased the number of punished licks in a Vogel conflict assay at doses ranging from 3 to 30 mg/kg. In a conditioned anxiety model in rats (conditioned lick suppression), a dose-dependent increase in licks was observed following suppression by tone paired with shock. Administration of **47** did not affect spontaneous

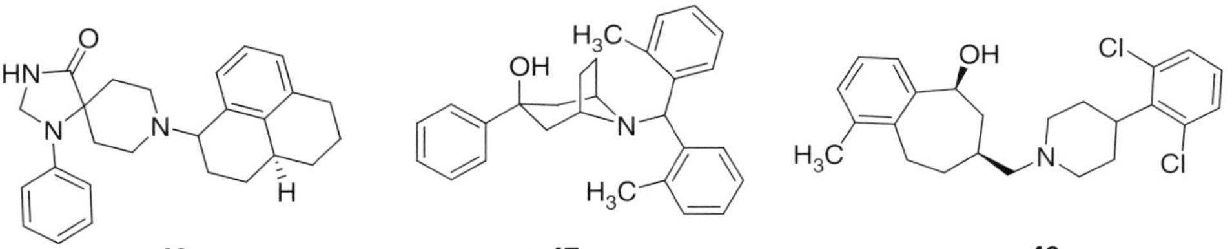

Figure 7.17 Structure of **46–48**.

locomotor activity or motor coordination over a dose range of 3–30 mg/kg. Furthermore, the effects of SCH 221510 were antagonized in the Vogel conflict model by the NOP-1 antagonist J-113397, indicating that the antidepressant activity was likely mediated by the NOP-1 receptor.

SB-612111 [64,65], **48**, a structurally distinct NOP-1 antagonist, was characterized in a similar series of in-vivo assays. In vitro, **48** showed a K_i value of 0.7 nM, and high selectivity versus other opioid receptors, and an EC_{50} of 0.7 nM. In anti-anxiety assays, the compound was administered intraperitoneally to mice in a forced swim test at 1, 3, and 10 mg/kg, and only the highest dose tested reduced immobility time. Administration of the endogenous peptide agonist N/OFQ by icv injection reversed this action. When **48** was tested in NOP-1 knockout mice, there was no effect on immobility time. There were no alterations in spontaneous locomotor activity when mice were treated with 10 mg/kg **48**.

The contrasting functional activity of these two molecules, and their in-vivo activity in preclinical assays predictive of antidepressant activity create a conundrum that will require additional investigation in order to ascertain this target's potential therapeutic utility.

Targets in the hypothalamic–pituitary–adrenal axis

The hypothalamic–pituitary–adrenal (HPA) axis is the body's major neuroendocrine system that is activated in response to stress. Dysfunction in the HPA axis has been established in both major depressive disorder and post-traumatic stress disorder [66,67]. In addition, treatment relapse in patients is associated with a disregulated HPA axis [68]. As a result, this system and its associated molecular targets, such as glucocorticoid, arginine vasopressin, and corticotropin-releasing factor (CRF) receptors are of interest for the development of anti-anxiety agents. This section will focus on glucocorticoid and vasopressin receptor developments in the last few years [69].

Glucocorticoid receptor antagonists

The endogenous glucocorticoid, cortisol, is well known to have an effect on CNS functions related to mood [70]. This action is exerted through glucocorticoid receptors (GR) that are widely distributed in the brain. Cortisol levels are elevated during periods of stress, and the steroid provides negative feedback regulation on the HPA axis [69]. In view of these data, recent reports suggest that GR antagonists exhibit activity in preclinical assays predictive of anxiolytic activity. In this field, it is important to establish not only binding affinity to the GR, it is also necessary to determine functional activity and selectivity for other nuclear hormone receptors such as the mineralocorticoid and progesterone receptors.

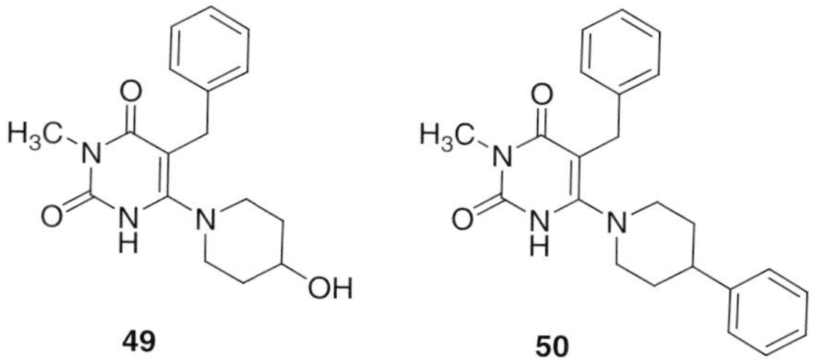

Figure 7.18 Structure of **49** and **50**.

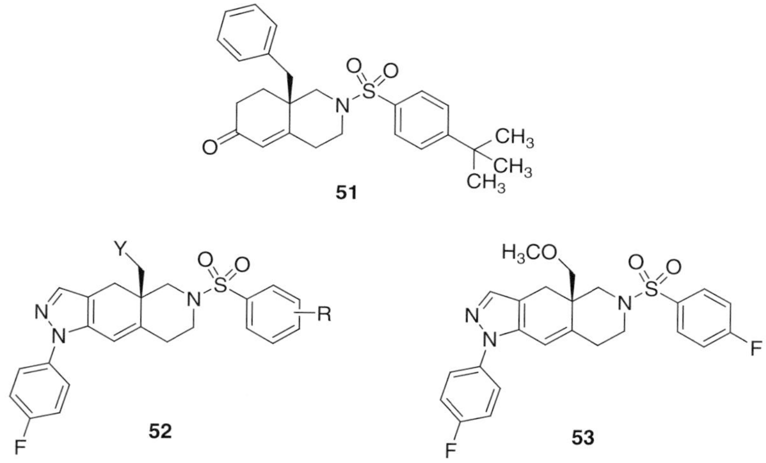

49

50

Figure 7.19 Structure of **51–53**.

51

52

53

Using a virtual screen, 3D similarity searches were conducted based on known GR antagonists. This resulted in the identification of a pyrimidinedione, **49** (Figure 7.18), a non-steroidal compound with a K_i value of 4.5 μM in a GR binding assay [71]. Subsequent optimization of this structure focused on modification of the piperidine ring, because similarity screening of related compounds suggested that changes in this region of the molecule improved GR affinity and functional activity. Structure–activity studies revealed that lipophilicity in this region of the molecule was important, and that replacement of the hydroxyl moiety in **49** with an unsubstituted phenyl ring, as in **50**, improved binding affinity and antagonist functional activity (binding K_i 8.1 nM, functional K_i 93 nM). Preliminary pharmaceutical property and pharmacokinetic evaluation revealed good metabolic stability, 25% inhibition of CYP3A4 at 1 μM, C_{max} of 143 ng/ml following a 5 mg/kg oral dose and a 1:4 brain/plasma ratio. Steroid receptor selectivity screening of compound **50** showed no affinity for the estrogen receptor, less than 50% binding at 1 μM to the progesterone and aldosterone receptors, and a K_i value of 930 nM at the mineralocorticoid receptor.

Clark and co-workers recently reported the discovery of pyrazolohexahydroisoquino-lines, **52**, that display high-affinity GR binding and functional antagonist activity. Selected compounds in this series also show evidence for brain penetration [72]. This series was derived from an azadecalinone template, **51**, where the pyrazole ring mimics the polarity of the ketone in **51** (Figure 7.19). The 4-fluorophenyl moiety on the pyrazole

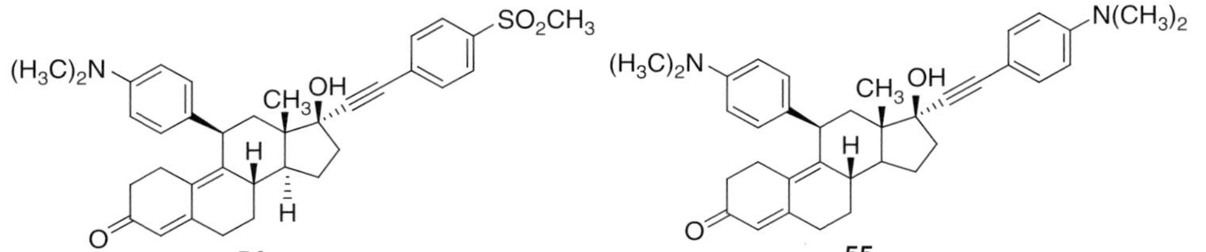

Figure 7.20 Structure of **54** and **55**.

was adopted as a standard, because this group was a key feature in the structure of known GR partial agonists [73]. A variety of aryl sulfonamide derivatives were prepared and studied, and many of these analogs showed high affinity (K_i < 30 nM), with variable antagonistic functional activity. Compound **53** (binding K_i 1.4 nM, antagonist K_i 33 nM) was evaluated in a pharmacokinetic screen, and showed 22% bioavailability in rats, with a brain:plasma ratio of 1.1:1. None of these pyrazole derivatives showed significant binding to other steroid receptors at concentrations up to 10 μM.

Studies with the GR antagonist ORG 34850, **54** (Figure 7.20), in rats suggest that prolonged blockade of the GR receptor is required before increased activity in the HPA axis can be observed [74]. This conclusion was based on the observation that cortisol levels increased after 5 days of treatment with 10 mg/kg of **54**, and no change in the level of the steroid hormone was seen in the 24 h following a single dose. The selective GR antagonist ORG 34116, **55**, was studied in a rat forced swim model for antidepressant activity [75]. The compound was administered at a dose of 20 mg/kg in the chow of rats for 4 weeks before the animals were subjected to the behavioral test. The data showed a significant reduction in immobility time compared to vehicle-treated animals. This positive result was coupled with increased phospho-CREB levels in the nuclei of dentate gyrus granular neurons and in the neocortex. In drug-treated animals, p-CREB levels decreased in both brain regions with time after the forced swim test.

Vasopressin receptor antagonists

Antagonism of the vasopressin 1B (V_{1B}) receptor is another potential approach for modulation of the HPA axis. In patients with melancholic or anxious-retarded depression, elevated levels of the endogenous ligand, arginine vasopressin, have been measured [76,77]. Additionally, an increase in the number of neurons that express the peptide in the brains of depressed patients has been measured [78]. SSR149415, **56** (Figure 7.21), has been widely used to study the role of V_{1B} receptors, their influence on the HPA axis, and to assess the potential of this target for the treatment of depression [79]. One potential drawback associated with the use of this compound is the observation that it also can antagonize oxytocin receptors [80]. In the original characterization of **56**, K_i values of 4.2 and 174 nM, respectively, for the human V_{1B} receptor and oxytocin receptor were reported [79]. Subsequently, Griffante and co-workers reported a K_i value of 0.5 nM at the V_{1B} receptor, and 2 nM at the oxytocin receptor [80].

SSR149415 was administered to olfactory bulbectomized rats at oral doses of 10 and 30 mg/kg orally acutely and chronically. Chronic (14 day) treatment reduced hyperemotionality in a dose-responsive manner; however, no effect was seen in the acute model [81]. The compound was also evaluated in a differential reinforcement of low rate

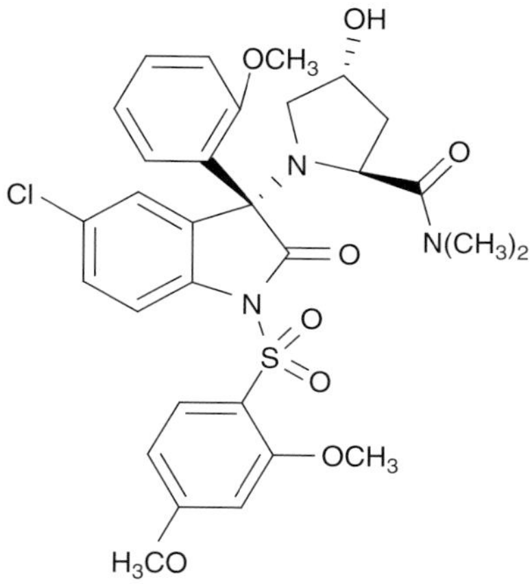

Figure 7.21 Structure of **56**.

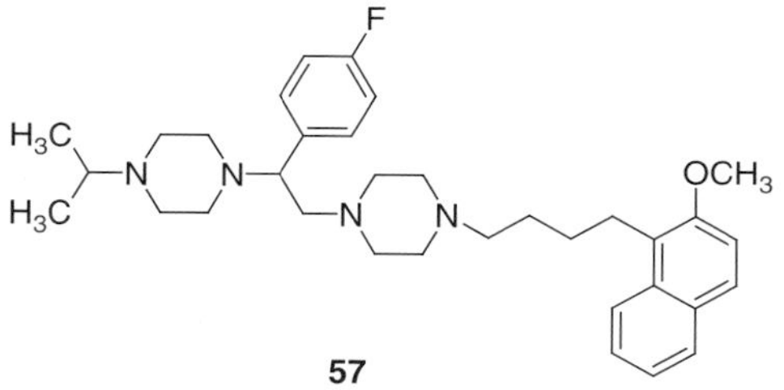

Figure 7.22 Structure of **57** and **58**.

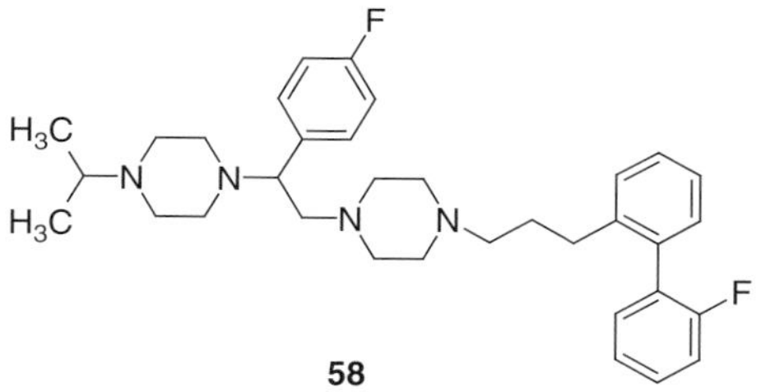

72s (DRL-72s) model in Wister rats that can be used to distinguish anxiolytic and antidepressant modes of action [82]. In this screen, **56** was administered ip at doses of 10 and 30 mg/kg, and in a dose-dependent manner increased the percentage of reinforced responses and shifted distribution curves toward longer duration. This profile was similar to the SSRI fluoxetine. For a more comprehensive summary of earlier in-vivo studies with SSR149415, see [69].

Melanocortin receptor antagonists

There are five known melanocortin (MC) receptor subtypes (1–5) that have been implicated in a wide range of physiologic functions. Unlike other receptors in the family, the MC4 receptor is found primarily in the central nervous system in brain regions associated with mood and emotion, including the amygdala, hippocampus, enthorhinal cortex, and hypothalamus [83,84]. This distribution suggests an association with the HPA axis. Endogenous ligands for the MC4 receptor, such as ACTH and α-MSH (melanin-stimulating hormone), are known to induce stress-related behavior in animals, such as excessive grooming [85]. In addition, electrical stress has been reported to increase expression of the MC4 receptor in the amygdala of rats [86].

Recent reports have demonstrated that non-peptide MC4 antagonists exhibit activity in a variety of antidepressant animal models. MCL0129, **57**, (MC4 IC_{50} 12.7 nM, Figure 7.22) was administered subcutaneously to rats in forced swim and learned helplessness behavioral assays. In the former, at doses of 3, 10, and 30 mg/kg, immobility time was reduced in a dose–response manner at the two higher doses. At doses of 1, 3, and 10 mg/kg in the learned helplessness model, both 3 and 10 mg/kg doses significantly reduced the number of escape failures, compared to vehicle-treated animals [87]. Structure–activity studies [88] on MCL0129 and analogs reveal that naphthalene and biphenyl moieties are well tolerated by the receptor. Interestingly, biphenyl derivatives display activity as inhibitors of dopamine reuptake as well as potent MC4 antagonism. A 2-substitutent on the naphthalene nucleus is important for high MC4 affinity, a 4-fluorophenyl moiety is preferred along the ethylene diamine chain between the two piperazine rings, and a three- or four-carbon linker between the biphenyl/naphthyl moiety and piperazine core is optimal. Compound 58 is an example of an MC4 agonist with dopamine reuptake inhibition activity.

Summary and outlook

Pharmacologic treatment for depression is now a well-recognized and accepted approach to assist patients with this disease. SSRIs and SNRIs are better tolerated than tricyclic antidepressants; however, as many as 30–40% of patients do not respond to these agents, and in some cases, side effects and delayed onset of activity are problematic [14]. As a result, there is considerable interest in other mechanisms to control mood, and these efforts have been aided by improved understanding of neurochemical pathways in key brain regions that influence mood and emotion. The potential targets and some of the molecules identified in this chapter are now being investigated clinically to validate the approach. Researchers in the field are continuing to work to develop new targets and treatment regimens that have the potential to address the perceived shortcomings associated with currently available agents. These new mechanisms go beyond monoamine-based therapies and include excitatory amino acids, neuropeptides, and endocrine pathways.

References

1. Kelly, J., *Curr. Med. Chem. Cent. Nerv. Syst. Agents*, 2003, **3**, 311.

2. Butler, S. G., Meegan, M. J. *Curr. Med. Chem.*, 2008, **15**, 1737.

3. Abramets, I. I., Evdokimov, D. V., Talalaenko, A. N., *Neurophysiology*, 2007, **39**, 184.

4. Demyttenaere, K., De Fruyt, J., Stahl, S. M., *Int. J. Neuropsychopharmacol.*, 2005, **8**, 93.

5. Katz, M. M., Tekell, J. L., Bowden, C. L., Brannan, S., Houston, J. P., Berman, N., *Neuropsychopharmacology*, 2004, **29**, 566.

6. Posternak, M. A., Zimmerman, M., *J. Clin. Psychiatry*, 2005, **66**, 148.

7. Blier, P., Montigny, C., *Biol. Psychiatry*, 1998, **44**, 213.

8. Manji, H. K., Chen, G., *Mol. Psychiatry*, 2002, **7**, S46.

9. Wong, M. L., Licinio, J., *Nat. Rev. Drug Discov.*, 2004, **3**, 136.

10. Xu, H., Richardson, J. S., Li, X. M., *Neuropsychopharmacology*, 2003, **28**, 53.

11. Gonul, A. S., Doksat, K., Eker, C., Eker, O. D., *Trends Serotonin Uptake Inhibitor Res*, 2005, 1.

12. Manji, H. K., Drevets, W. C., Charney, D. S., *Nat. Med.*, 2001, **7**, 541.

13. Coyle, J. T., Duman, R. S., *Neuron*, 2003, **38**, 157.

14. Rosenzweig-Lipson, S., Beyer, C. E., Hughes, Z., et al., *Pharmacol. Ther.*, 2007, **113**, 134.

15. Cipriani, A., Barbui, C., Brambilla, P., Furukawa, T. A., Hotopf, M., Geddes, J. R., *J. Clin. Psychiatry*, 2006, **67**, 850.

16. Thase, M. E., *J. Clin. Psychiatry*, 1998, **59**, 502.

17. DeMontigny, C., Chaput, I., Blier, P., *J. Clin. Psychopharmacol.*, 1987, **7**, 24.

18. Romero, L., Hervás, I., Artegas, F., *Neurosci. Lett.*, 1996, **219**, 123.

19. Duxon, M. S., Starr, K. R., Upton, N., *Br. J. Pharmacol.*, 2000, **130**, 1713.

20. Takeuchi, K., Kohn, T. J., Honigschmidt, N. A., et al., *Bioorg. Med. Chem. Lett.*, 2003, **13**, 1903.

21. Takeuchi, K., Kohn, T. J., Honigschmidt, N. A., et al., *Bioorg. Med. Chem. Lett.*, 2006, **16**, 2347.

22. Hatzenbuhler, N. T., Evrard, D. A., Harrison, B. L., et al., *J. Med. Chem.*, 2006, **49**, 4785.

23. Hatzenbuhler, N. T., Baudy, R., Evrard, D. A., et al., *J. Med. Chem.*, 2008, **51**, 6980.

24. Kreiss, D. S., Lucki, I., *J. Pharmacol. Exp. Ther.*, 1995, **274**, 866.

25. Atkinson, P. J., Bromidge, S. M., Duxon, M. S., et al., *Bioorg. Med. Chem. Lett.*, 2005, **15**, 737.

26. Scott, C., Soffin, E. M., Hill, M., et al., *Eur. J. Pharmacol.*, 2006, **536**, 54.

27. Starr, K. R., Price, G. W., Watson, J. M., et al., *Neuropsychopharmacology*, 2007, **32**, 2163.

28. Skolnick, P., Popik, P, Janowsky, A., Beer, B., Lippa, A. S., *Eur. J. Pharmacol.*, 2003, **461**, 99.

29. D'Aquila, P. S., Collu, M., Gessa, G. L., Serra, G., *Eur. J. Pharmacol.*, 2000, **405**, 365.

30. Naranjo, C., Tremblay, L. K., Busto, U. E., *Prog. Neuropsychopharmacol. Biol. Psychiatry*, 2001, **25**, 781.

31. Skolnick, P., Popik, P., Janowsky, A., Beer, B., Lippa, A. S., *Life Sci.*, 2003, **73**, 3175.

32. Ben-Jonathan, N., Hnasko, R., *Endocr. Rev.*, 2001, **22**, 724.

33. Breuer, M. E., Chan, J. S. W., Oosting, R. S., et al., *Eur. Neuropsychopharmacol.*, 2008, **18**, 908.

34. Carlier, P. R., Lo, M. M., Lo, P. C., et al., *Bioorg. Med. Chem. Lett.*, 1998, **8**, 487.

35. Liang, Y., Shaw, A. M., Boules, M., et al., *J. Pharmacol. Exp. Ther.*, 2008, **327**, 573.

36. Aluisio, L., Lord, B., Barbier, A., et al., *Eur. J. Pharmacol.*, 2008, **587**, 141.

37. Bannwart, L. M., Carter, D. S., Cai, H. Y., et al., *Bioorg. Med. Chem. Lett.*, 2008, **18**, 6062.

38. Trullas, R., Skolnick, P., *Eur. J. Pharmacol.*, 1990, **185**, 1.

39. Paul, I. A., Layer, R. T., Skolnick, P, Nowak, G., *Eur. J. Pharmacol.*, 1993, **247**, 305.

40. Paul, I. A., Nowak, G., Layer, R. T., Skolnick, P., *J. Pharmacol. Exp. Ther.*, 1994, **269**, 95.

41. Nowak, G., Legutko, B., Skolnick, P., Popik, P., *Eur. J. Pharmacol.*, 1998, **342**, 367.

42. Zarate, C. A., Singh, J. B., Carlson, P. J., et al., *Arch. Gen. Psychiatry*, 2006, **63**, 856.

43. Pilc, A., Chaki, S., Nowak, G., Witkin, J. M., *Biochem. Pharmacol.*, 2008, **75**, 997.

44. Lea, P. M., Faden, A. I., *CNS Drug Rev.*, 2006, **12**, 149.

45. Li, X., Need, A. B., Baez, M., Witkin, J. M., *J. Pharmacol. Exp. Ther.*, 2006, **319**, 254.

46. Sharma, S., Rodriguez, A. L., Conn, J. P., Lindsley, C. W., *Bioorg. Med. Chem. Lett.*, 2008, **18**, 4098.

47. Porter, R. H. P., Jaeschke, G., Spooren, W., et al., *J. Pharmacol. Exp. Ther.*, 2005, **315**, 711.

48. Rodriguez, A. L., Nong, Y., Sekaran, N. K., Alagille, D., Tamagnan, G. D., Conn, P. J., *Mol. Pharmacol.*, 2005, **68**, 793.

49. Milbank, J. B. J., Knauer, C. S., Augelli-Szafran, C. E., et al., *Bioorg. Med. Chem. Lett.*, 2007, **17**, 4415.

50. Bach, P., Nilsson, K., Svensson, T., et al., *Bioorg. Med. Chem. Lett.*, 2006, **16**, 4788.

51. Ohishi, H., Shigemoto, R., Nakanishi, S., Mizuno, N., *Neuroscience*, 1993, **53**, 1009.

52. Tanabe, Y., Nomura, A., Masu, M., Shigemoto, R., Mizuno, N., *J. Neurosci.*, 1993, **13**, 1372.

53. Shigemoto, R., Kinoshita, A., Wada, E., et al., *J. Neurosci.*, 1997, **17**, 7503.

54. Ohishi, H., Shigemoto, R., Nakanishi, S., Mizuno, N., *J. Comp. Neurol.*, 1993, **335**, 252.

55. Spinelli, S., Ballard, T., Gatti-McArthur, S., et al., *Psychopharmacology*, 2005, **179**, 292.

56. Higgins, G. A., Ballard, T. M., Kew, J. N. C., et al., *Neuropharmacology*, 2004, **46**, 907.

57. Woltering, T. J., Adam, G., Alanine, A., et al., *Bioorg. Med. Chem. Lett.*, 2007, **17**, 6811.

58. Woltering, T. J., Adam, G., Wichmann, J., et al., *Bioorg. Med. Chem. Lett.*, 2008, **18**, 1091.

59. Nakazato, A., Sakagami, K., Yasuhara, A., et al., *J. Med. Chem.*, 2004, **47**, 4570.

60. Yasuhara, A., Nakamura, M., Sakagami, K., et al., *Bioorg. Med. Chem.*, 2006, **14**, 4193.

61. Reinschied, R., *CNS Neurol Disord Drug Targets*, 2006, **5**, 219.

62. Jenck, F., Wichmann, J., Dautzenberg, F. M., et al., *Proc. Natl Acad. Sci.*, 2000, **97**, 4938.

63. Varty, G. B., Lu, S. X., Morgan, C. A., et al., *J. Pharmacol. Exp. Ther.*, 2008, **326**, 672.

64. Spagnolo, B., Carrà, G., Fantin, M., et al., *J. Pharmacol. Exp. Ther.*, 2007, **321**, 961.

65. Rizzi, A., Gavioli, E. C., Marzola, G., et al., *J. Pharmacol. Exp. Ther.*, 2007, **321**, 968.

66. Schatzberg, A. F., Rothschild, A. J., Langlais, P. J., Bird, E. D., Cole, J. O., *J. Psychiatr. Res.*, 1985, **19**, 57.

67. Marshall, R. D., Blanco, C., Printz, D., Liebowitz, M. R., Klein, D. F., Coplan, J., *Psychiatry Res.*, 2002, **110**, 219.

68. Zobel, A. W., Nickel, T., Sonntag, A., Uhr, M., Holsboer, F., Ising, M., *J. Psychiatr. Res.*, 2001, **35**, 83.

69. Thomson, F., Craighead, M., *Neurochem. Res.*, 2008, **33**, 691.

70. Erickson, K., Drevets, W., Schulkin, J., *Neurosci. Biobehav. Rev.*, 2003, **27**, 233.

71. Ray, N. C., Clark, R. D., Clark, D. E., et al., *Bioorg. Med. Chem. Lett.*, 2007, **17**, 4901.

72. Clark, R. D., Ray, N. C., Williams, K., et al., *Bioorg. Med. Chem. Lett.*, 2008, **18**, 1312.

73. Shah, N., Scanlan, T., *Bioorg. Med. Chem. Lett.*, 2004, **14**, 5199.

74. Spiga, F., Harrison, L. R., Wood, S. A., et al., *J. Neuroendocrinology*, 2007, **19**, 891.

75. Bachmann, C. G., Bilang-Bleuel, A., De Carli, S., Linthorst, A. C. E., Reul, J. M. H. M., *Neuroendocrinology*, 2005, **81**, 129.

76. de Winter, R. F., van Hemert, A. M., DeRijk, R. H., et al., *Neuropsychopharmacology*, 2003, **28**, 140.

77. van Londen, L., Goekoop, J. G., van Kempen, G. M., et al., *Neuropsychopharmacology*, 1993, **17**, 284

78. Purba, J. S., Hoogendijk, W. J., Hofman, M. A., Swaab, D. F., *Arch. Gen. Psychiatry*, 1996, **53**, 137.

79. Serradeil-Le Gal, C., Wagnon, J., Simiand, J., et al., *J. Pharmacol. Exp. Ther.*, 2002, **300**, 1122.

80. Griffante, C., Green, A., Curcuruto, O., Haslam, C. P., Dickinson, B. A., Arban, R., *Br. J. Pharmacol.*, 2005, **146**, 744.

81. Iijima, M., Chaki, S., *Prog. Neuropsychopharmacol. Biol. Psych.*, 2007, **31**, 622.

82. Louis, C., Cohen, C., Depoortére, R., Griebel, R., *Neuropsychopharmacology*, 2006, **31**, 2180.

83. Mountjoy, K. G., Mortrud, M. T., Low, M. J., Simerly, R. B., Cone, R. D., *Mol. Endocrinol.* 1994, **8**, 1298.

84. Chhajlani, V., *Biochem. Mol. Biol. Int.*, 1996, **38**, 73.

85. Adan, R. A., Szklarczyk, A. W., Oosterom, J., et al., *Eur. J. Pharmacol.*, 1999, **378**, 249.

86. Yamano, Y., Yoshioka, M., Toda, Y., et al., *J. Vet. Med. Sci.*, 2004, **66**, 1323.

87. Chaki, S., Hirota, S., Funakoshi, T., et al., *J. Pharmacol. Exp. Ther.*, 2003, **304**, 818.

88. Nozawa, D., Okubo, T., Ishii, T., et al., *Bioorg. Med. Chem.*, 2007, **15**, 1989.

Application of pharmacogenomics and personalized medicine for the care of depression

Keh-Ming Lin, Chun-Yu Chen, and Yu-Jui Yvonne Wan

Abstract

Remarkable progress notwithstanding, pharmacotherapy for depressive and related conditions, as well as pharmacological intervention of various other psychiatric and medical conditions, has typically ignored the magnitude and clinical relevance of the huge inter-individual variations in pharmacokinetics and pharmacodynamics. Such neglects lead to additional risks of severe and/or unpleasant side effects, medication non-adherence, prolonged periods of titration, suboptimal therapeutic responses, and treatment failures. Advances in pharmacogenomics and computer modeling technologies hold promises for achieving the goals of "personalized" ("individualized") medicine. However, challenges abound for realizing such goals, including the packaging and interpretation of genotyping results, ethical considerations, financing, economy of scale, inertia against changes in medical practice (innovation diffusion), as well as other infrastructural and organizational issues related to the use of new information.

Introduction

In the context of the rapidly expanding knowledge base and revolutionizing progress in the field of psychopharmacology, and pharmacotherapy in general, terms such as "personalized" or "individualized" medicines appear oxymoronic [1–5]. This notwithstanding, current pharmacological practices continue to ignore or minimize individual and cross-group variations, which often are extremely sizable. Textbooks and package inserts provided by pharmaceutical companies give a fairly narrow range for dosing recommendations. Consequently, medications initially prescribed for many patients may not be the optimal choices for them, and the dosing may be many magnitudes lower than required. Yet for equally substantial proportions of patients, "regular" dosing as initially prescribed may be grossly excessive. Also, there is currently no rational bases for choosing one class or type of medication over the other (e.g. selective serotonin uptake inhibitors vs. others). This "one size fits all" approach is often the reason for poor treatment response, non-adherence, severe and at times potentially fatal side effects, and unnecessary hospitalization. Pharmacogenetics and pharmacogenomics (PG) hold great promise for addressing these issues. This appears particularly ironic, since, with the insight and impressive knowledge base already accumulated over the past several decades, a great deal is already known about factors governing both

Next Generation Antidepressants: Moving Beyond Monoamines to Discover Novel Treatment Strategies for Mood Disorders, ed. Chad E. Beyer and Stephen M. Stahl. Published by Cambridge University Press.
© Cambridge University Press 2010.

the pharmacokinetics and pharmacodynamics of most drugs, and the technology is largely there to put these advances into clinical use. With the field continuing to progress at lightening speed, such a proposition will become increasingly self-evident.

Such apparent discrepancies between the progress of PG on the one hand and its clinical application on the other may be largely the consequence of a number of major obstacles that will continue to prevent the bridging of such gaps without major efforts to overcome them. These include (1) feasibility of incorporating PG input (CPG) in clinical decision making, and the impact of such an approach on clinical outcome and cost-effectiveness analyses [6–8]; (2) complexity and apparent "over-abundance" of PG information vis-à-vis drug response; (3) inherent "inertia" hindering the "diffusion of innovation," and the need for incorporating PG approaches in medical education [9]; (4) problems related to the "economy of scale"; and financial support for new approaches [10]; (5) ethical concerns [11], including worries about privacy [12], equality of the use of healthcare resources [13], and misuse of genetic information.

In the following, we will briefly review the literature suggesting that CPG is feasible and clinically relevant; that depressed subjects treated with the CPG approach will show significantly less side effects (greater tolerability), greater medication adherence, better clinical outcome, and a lower rate of relapse. Such data should be encouraging for medical educators and policymakers in moving towards a broader adaptation of CPG as part of the standard of care, and the realization of the goals of what have been generally called "individualized" or "personalized" medicine.

The prevalence and health consequence of depressive problems

Numerous clinical and epidemiological studies, conducted over the past several decades, consistently indicate that clinically significant depression is a highly prevalent condition. For example, using the Composite International Diagnostic Interview (CIDI), the National Comorbid Study (NCS) found that up to 25% of the general population in the USA are at risk for DSM-III-R defined major depression at least once during their lifetime [14]. Utilizing similarly sophisticated research designs and assessment instruments, many well-designed studies have also been conducted in other countries, ranging from France to Korea [15]. Together, these studies clearly demonstrate that depression is a worldwide phenomenon, and is a serious public health threat in any society [16].

Approximately 15% of the people with the diagnosis of major depression eventually end their lives with suicide [17], making suicide one of the top ten causes of death in many countries in recent years. Recent studies also have documented the role depression plays in causing significant morbidity and functional impairment, resulting in substantial financial costs to society comparable to, or surpassing, many other relatively common medical problems, such as hypertension or diabetes [18]. Depression is also a major risk factor for many other life-threatening medical conditions, such as heart attacks, stroke, and cancers [19,20]. Furthermore, although acute depressive episodes are often time-limited, recent longitudinal follow-up studies show that relapses are often the rule rather than the exception, rendering the long-term outcome of such a condition far more ominous. Remission is often incomplete; many continue to suffer from subsyndromal depressive conditions, which have also been shown to be associated with significant functional disability [21,22].

Current status of antidepressant treatment: success and limitations

Since the 1950s, a large number of antidepressants (ADs) have been developed, each with proven efficacy in well-designed, placebo-controlled, randomized clinical trials. Starting with the classical tricyclic antidepressants and monoamine oxidase inhibitors, now clinicians also have a large array of newer antidepressants at their disposal, including the selective serotonin reuptake inhibitors, the serotonin–norepinephrine reuptake inhibitors, as well as a number of other "novel" antidepressants. These compounds, each with its unique profile, together afford clinicians with powerful tools in their attempts to bring patients back from the brink of despair. At the same time, the multiplicity and complexity presented by these diverse agents represent a puzzling challenge for clinicians both young and seasoned. Despite decades of research, it remains unclear why, despite their proven efficacy (with proven superiority compared to placebos), a relatively large proportion of the patients fail to respond to these agents, and why different patients might respond to different agents. In other words, there is at present no reliable method for clinicians to predict, prior to the initiation of treatment, which of the several dozens of ADs might be the best for the particular patient in the office. This plight is further worsened by the fact that there is a significant lag time, up to 4–6 weeks, before the full benefit of the medication could be assessed. Thus, for each "failed" treatment, substantive and often critical time is lost, leading at times to dire consequences including further aggravation, dropping-out due to side effects or disappointments regarding the lack of effects, which further increase the risk of mortality and worsening or persistent morbidity.

Similarly, clinicians currently have few means for determining the optimal starting dose for any of the ADs as prescribed for each individual patient. This is so despite the fact that huge inter-individual variations (up to 100 times) have been demonstrated for most, if not all, ADs (and most of the other medications, psychiatric and non-psychiatric). For a substantive proportion (usually about one-third) of the patients, the "standard" initial doses (as suggested in package inserts and in textbooks) represent only a small fraction of the optimal dose needed to achieve therapeutic effects. Yet for a similarly substantive proportion of the other patients, the "standard" initial doses lead to severe side effects. Further, the titration is essentially "trial and error," time-consuming, and contributes further to the delay in treatment response and recovery. Although the determination of the concentration of drugs and their metabolites in bodily fluids (typically with plasma or serum) could be useful in this regard [23–26], it is usually not available in clinical settings (it is unreasonable to expect clinical laboratories to have the capacity for measuring the "blood levels" of various ADs and their active metabolites, and to do it in a timely manner useful for clinical decision, i.e. a short turn-around time), and is typically done at steady state, requiring patients to be on a particular medication for an extended period of time before the measurement.

Thus, although ADs are efficacious, neither their choice nor the dosing strategy are based on rational principles, leading to substantial "false starts," delay in response, diminished medication adherence, "under- or over-treatment," iatrogenic problems, morbidity, and even mortality.

The promise of pharmacogenetics/pharmacogenomics

In such a context, it is even more alarming that knowledge derived from the field of pharmacogenetics/pharmacogenomics has not yet made inroads into enhancing clinicians' ability to "individualize" or "personalize" pharmacotherapy. Evolving over the past half century, the field of pharmacogenetics has provided the basis for our understanding of many "idiosyncratic" drug reactions [27]. In recent years, it elucidated much of the genetic basis of individual variations in pharmacokinetics (especially genes determining drug metabolism) and pharmacodynamics (therapeutic target responses) [28,29]. Their relevance for ADs is summarized below:

Genes encoding enzymes and other protein products responsible for the fate and disposition of psychotropics (pharmacokinetics) (Table 8.1)

As is true with many other pharmacological agents, the biotransformation of practically all ADs are primarily mediated by a group of enzymes called cytochrome P-450 enzymes (CYPs) including CYP2D6, CYP2C19, CYP2C9, CYP3As, and CYP1A2. Huge individual variations in the activities of these enzymes have long been demonstrated, much of which have been accounted for with specific allelic variations in the genes encoding these enzymes [30]. For example, CYP2D6 allelic profiles determine whether a particular individual is a poor metabolizer (those with defective genes encoding no enzyme; approximately 7% in Caucasians and less than 2% in East Asians), intermediate metabolizer (those with "less effective" genes; approximately 50% in East Asians, caused by a genetic variant classified as CYP2D6*10; 30% in those with sub-Saharan African ancestry due to a different variant classified as CYP2D6*17), extensive metabolizer (those with "wild-type" alleles; approximately 90% in Caucasians and 47% in East Asians), and ultra-rapid metabolizer (those with gene duplication or multiplication; in Caucasians the prevalence of such a variant ranges from 1% to 5%; in Ethiopians, Arabians, and Sephardic Jews the prevalence is significantly

Table 8.1 Candidate genes and corresponding SNP densities (pharmacokinetics)

Gene	Gene name	Chromosomal location	Size (bp)	Public database SNPs	
				# SNPs	Mean distance between SNPs (kb)
Cytochrome P450 1A2	CYP1A2	15q24.1	7 776	28	0.6
Cytochrome P450 2C19C	CYP2C19	10q23.33	90 209	31	3.2
Cytochrome P450 2D6	CYP2D6	22q13.1	14 797	125	0.1
Cytochrome P450 3A4	CYP3A4	7q22.1	27 205	66	0.7
Cytochrome P450 3A5	CYP3A5	7q22.1	31 790	15	2.7
Constitutive androstane receptor	CAR, NR1I3	1q21.3	8 511	28	0.3
Steroid and xenobiotic recepter	SXR, NR1I2	3q12-q13.3	38 001	69	0.6
Orosomucoid 1	ORM1	9q32	3 422	70	0.3
Orosomucoid 2	ORM2	9q32	3 230	73	0.3
Multiple drug resistance 1	MDR1	7q21.1	209 390	202	1.0
UDP-glycosyltransferase	UGT2B7	4q13.2	16 451	0	0
UDP-glycosyltransferase	UGT2B15	4q13.2	23 987	46	0.9

higher, ranging up to 29%) [31–35]. Studies involving desipramine and venlafaxine clearly indicate that these CYP2D6 polymorphisms are mainly responsible for the pharmacokinetics, dosing, and side effect profiles of these CYP2D6 substrates [36,37]. Similarly, specific allelic alterations also have been demonstrated to determine CYP2C19 enzyme activities, and consequently the dosing and side effect profiles of medications metabolized by this enzyme [38–40]. In addition, the activity of some of these CYPs also could be significantly altered by exposure to environmental agents, whose mechanisms also have been elucidated. For example, the induction effect of St. John's wort (and other natural substances) on CYP3A4 is now known to be mediated via the steroid and xenobiotic receptor (SXR), and the induction of CYP1A2 by constituents of cigarettes is mediated through the activation of the Ah receptor [41].

Although less well-documented, a number of genes other than the CYPs also influence the process of pharmacokinetics, and thus are also likely to affect the dosing and side-effect profiles of ADs. These include genes encoding transferases, such as glutathione-S-transferase (GST) and UDP-glucuronosyltransferases (UGTs), which are responsible for drug conjugation; multidrug-resistance gene (MDR1) encoding the P-glycoprotein responsible for exporting lipophilic compounds to the extracellular space (and thus reducing drug absorption in the gut as well as inhibiting their crossing the blood–brain barrier) [42,43]; and orosomucoid 1 and 2 (ORM1 and ORM2) encoding the alpha$_1$ acid glycoproteins responsible for the binding of psychotropics to plasma proteins, which is often extensive [44,45].

Genes encoding therapeutic targets of ADs (pharmacodynamics) (Table 8.2)

A number of monoamine neurotransmitter systems, including 5-HT, NE, and DA, may all play crucial roles in mediating vulnerability to depressive disorders [46–48]. Moreover, most of the commonly prescribed antidepressants are believed to exert their effects at least in part through the modulation of either the 5-HT or the NE systems, or both [47,48]. As the proximal site of action of many antidepressants in clinical use, the genes modulating the 5-HT, NE, and DA systems therefore represent attractive functional candidates in exploring antidepressant response. Each of these systems is influenced by three types of gene products: (1) those involved in biosynthesis and catabolism of the monoamines; (2) those encoding receptors mediating their effects; and (3) those encoding specific transporters responsible for removing them from the synapses [46]. Although a large number of studies have been conducted examining the association between many of these genes and antidepressant response as well as risk for mood and associated disorders, results have often been inconsistent. Of these, however, the serotonin transporter (SERT or 5-HTT) appears most promising. As the target of SSRIs, 5-HTT clearly plays a crucial role in determining patients' response to these antidepressants, and thus it is reasonable to speculate that functional genetic polymorphism(s) should bear clinical relevance. This indeed appears to be the case with the 5-HTT gene-linked polymorphic region (5-HTTLPR), a 44 base-pair insertion/deletion in the promoter region, which significantly influences the basal transcriptional activity of 5-HTT [49], resulting in differential 5-HTT expression and 5-HT cellular uptake [50]. Hariri et al. [51] reported that subjects who are homozygotic for the l allele for 5-HTTLPR showed less fear and anxiety-related behaviors and exhibited less amygdala neuronal

Table 8.2 Candidate genes and corresponding SNP densities (pharmacodynamics/signaling)

Gene	Gene name	Chromosomal location	Size (bp)	Public database SNPs	
				# SNPs	Mean distance between SNPs (kb)
5-HT genes					
* Serotonin 1A receptor	HTR1A	5q12.3	1 269	12	0.8
* Serotonin 2A receptor	HTR2A	13q14.2	62 661	121	0.6
* Serotonin 2C receptor	HTR2C	Xq24	326 074	147	2.3
* Serotonin transporter	HTT SLC6A4	17q11.2	24 118	33	1.1
* Tryptophan hydroxylase	TPH	11p15.1	19 772	53	0.8
NE/DA genes					
* Monoamine oxidase A	MAOA	X-p11.3	70 206	51	1.7
* Catechol-O-methyl transferase	COMT	22q11.21	27 135	91	0.4
* Adrenergic alpha2A receptor	ADRA2A	10q25.2	36 50	22	0.9
* Norepinephrine transporter	NET1 SLC6A2	16q12.2	46 031	122	0.5
* Dopamine D2 receptor iso l/s	DRD2	11q23.2	65 577	98	0.8
* Dopamine D3 receptor iso a-d	DRD3	3q13.31	50 200	73	0.9
* Dopamine D4 receptor	DRD4	11p15.5	3 400	20	0.6
* Dopamine D5 receptor	DRD5	4p16.1	2 032	48	0.4
* Dopamine transporter	DAT SLC6A3	5p15.33	52 637	337	0.2
Other novel loci (example)					
* Brain-derived neurotrophic factor	BDNF	11p14.1	42 903	30	2.0

activity as assessed by functional MRI in response to fearful stimuli. In congruence with this, a large number of studies have suggested association between this polymorphism and anxiety, depression, and suicide risks. The relationship between 5-HTTLPR polymorphisms and antidepressant response has been intriguing. Seven of nine studies [52–60], including one from Taiwan [52], showed that the 5-HTTLPR l allele is associated with better or more rapid SSRI response. Two recent studies also implicate the 5-HTTLPR s allele in SSRI-emergent adverse effects [61,62]. Interestingly, 5-HTTLPR genotype polymorphism also exhibits remarkable cross-ethnic variations [63], which is the case with the majority of the genes encoding therapeutic targets of ADs and other psychotropics as well.

Other genes that have been the target of similar investigations include serotonin 2A receptor (5-HT2A) [64–67], dopamine transporter (DAT1) [68–75], dopamine D2, D3, D4 receptor (DRD2, DRD3, DRD4), norepinephrine transporter (NET), adrenalin 2A receptor (ADRA2A) [76–79], beta adrenalin receptor (betaARs) [80], catechol-O-methyltransferase (COMT) [81], monoamine oxidase (MAO) [82–84], tryptophan hydroxylase (TPH) [55,85,86], G-protein beta3-subunit (Gbeta3) [87], apolipoprotein E epsilon4 [88], and brain-derived neurotrophic factor (BDNF) [89].

From pharmacogenomics to individualized medicine

Remarkable advances as described above notwithstanding, the goal of achieving "individualized medicine" remain elusive. Although part of this apparent lack of progress in the clinical application of pharmacogenomics may be attributable to existing gaps in the knowledge base, there is a general belief that the field has progressed to a point that sufficient information has already been accumulated that is clinically applicable. Some of the factors impeding the progress in this direction have to do with deficiency infrastructure as well as the sparsity of data showing efficacy and cost-effectiveness of the pharmacogenomic approach. In order to bridge these serious knowledge gaps and to move the field forward, towards clinical applications of pharmacogenomic principles, the authors suggest the following.

Development of pharmacogenomic panel(s)

Although for some drug-metabolizing enzymes, such as CYP2D6 and CYP2C19, allelic variations could lead to dramatic functional and health consequences, in the majority of the "candidate genes" for antidepressant response, the influence is partial and maybe accumulative. This means that many genes may influence treatment response, but each with only a small effect. This is especially true with genes encoding potential therapeutic targets. Although this has been the consensus in the field for a number of years, the extant pharmacogenetic literature is predominantly based on a single genotype or a combination of only a few genotypes. In order for pharmacogenetic data to be clinically useful, multiple relevant genotypes need to be tested simultaneously, and the results need to be available for clinicians in a timely manner (preferably within 24 h), such that the data could be included in the clinical decisions made prior to the initiation of pharmacotherapy. With the advent of high throughput genotyping technologies, this is no longer out of reach. Thus, the next generation of pharmacogenomic research should include the development of specific pharmacogenomic panel(s) for different disease categories and treatment methods.

Developing user-friendly tools for interpreting pharmacogenomic results

Since for any disease/treatment category, such a panel will likely include a large number of "candidate genes," whose function likely is influenced by multiple alleles, the results of the panel will be exceedingly complex and may not be easily interpretable by typical clinicians, much less readily incorporated into the clinical decision-making process. To solve such a problem, a number of modeling programs have been developed. Of these, the most promising appears to be the neural network and neural fuzzy models [90–93]. Using such a model, relevant genetic data as well as clinical, sociodemographic, and lifestyle variables (past medication response history, concurrent use of other medications, dietary practices, and exposure to other drug-inducing or inhibiting agents, such as cigarette smoking) could be incorporated simultaneously in the estimations for the probability of efficacy and dosing strategy for different medications. Further, a unique feature of such a model is that it is "trainable," in that as additional relevant data become available, they could be readily incorporated to improve the prediction model.

Pilot intervention project for clinical pharmacogenomics

Once established, such a therapeutic management system (pharmacogenomic panel and the interpreting tool) should then be examined in a series of studies to systematically examine its feasibility, acceptability, effectiveness, and ultimately cost-effectiveness. Randomized controlled trials could be designed with consenting subjects randomly assigned to experimental (pharmacogenomically informed) and control (decision based on current best practice guidelines).

There is little doubt that, while essential, the results of the studies as proposed would not be sufficient to bring "personalized" medicine to the level of routine clinical care. Many other non-technological factors as discussed earlier, commonly labeled as ethical, legal, and social implications (ELSI), as well as issues related to problems of economy of scales, funding, education, and innovation diffusion, also need to be tackled before the such goals could be realized [13,94]. However, any lingering uncertainties regarding the effectiveness (not just efficacy) of the pharmacogenomic approach would make these important dialogues exceedingly difficult.

Summary

In the past decade, the field of pharmacogenomics has exploded, resulting in a huge body of literature pointing to its promising and imminent clinical application and the realization of the goal of individualizing medical care. That this has not yet taken place is in all likelihood much less related to the incompleteness of information than to the absence of infrastructure such as the management system discussed above, and consequently the kind of intervention studies examining the clinical utility and cost-effectiveness of such an approach. While the more traditional association studies are still needed to further expand our knowledge base, it is timely that the field starts to explore ways to package knowledge that is already available, and examine their clinical application in well-designed studies. This represents an initial effort in this direction, with the goal of enhancing efficacy, reducing iatrogenic casualties, relieving untoward effects and suffering secondary to delayed treatment response, and ultimately, saving of medical care costs. This may lead to a major breakthrough in understanding with potential for radically changing the way medicine is practiced.

References

1. Fierz W. 2004, Challenge of personalized health care: to what extent is medicine already individualized and what are the future trends, *Med. Sci. Monit.*, **10**(5): 111.

2. Hallworth M. 2004, The drugs don't work: pharmacogenomics – clinical biochemistry's future? *Ann. Clin. Biochem.*, **41**(Pt 4): 260.

3. Ross J., Schenkein D., Kashala O., et al. 2004, Pharmacogenomics, *Adv. Anat. Pathol.*, **11**(4): 211.

4. Haga S. B., Burke W. 2004, Using pharmacogenetics to improve drug safety and efficacy, *JAMA*, **291**(23): 2869.

5. Lin K.-M., Perlis R. H., Wan Y.-J. 2008, Pharmacogenomic strategy for individualizing antidepressant therapy, *Dialogues Clin. Neurosci.*, **10**(4): 401.

6. Bala M., Zarkin G. 2004, Pharmacogenomics and the evolution of healthcare: is it time for cost-effectiveness

analysis at the individual level? *Pharmacoeconomics*, **22**(8): 495.

7. Evans W., Relling M. 2004, Moving towards individualized medicine with pharmacogenomics, *Nature*, **429**: 464.

8. Flowers C., Veenstra D. 2004, The role of cost-effectiveness analysis in the era of pharmacogenomics, *Pharmacoeconomics*, **22**(8): 481.

9. Frueh F., Gurwitz D. 2004, From pharmacogenetics to personalized medicine: a vital need for educating health professionals and the community, *Pharmacogenomics*, **5**(5): 571.

10. Phillips K., Veenstra D., Ramsey S., Van Bebber S., Sakowski J. 2004, Genetic testing and pharmacogenomics: issues for determining the impact to healthcare delivery and costs, *Am. J. Manag. Care*, **10**(7): 425.

11. Mordini E. 2004, Ethical considerations on pharmacogenomics, *Pharmacol. Res.*, **49**(4): 375.

12. Lin Z., Owen A., Altman R. 2004, Genetics: genomic research and human subject privacy, *Science*, **305**(5681): 183.

13. Voelter-Mahlknecht S., Mahlknecht U. 2004, Darwinism and pharmacogenomics: from 'one treatment fits all' to 'selection of the richest'? *Trends Mol. Med.*, **10**(5): 208.

14. Kessler R. C., McGonagle K. A., Zhao S., et al. 1994, Lifetime and 12-month prevalence of DSM-III-R psychiatric disorders in the United States. Results from the National Comorbidity Survey, *Arch. Gen. Psychiatry*, **51**(1): 8.

15. Weissman M. M., Bland R. C., Canino G. J., et al. 1996, Cross-national epidemiology of major depression and bipolar disorder, *JAMA*, **276**(4): 293.

16. Desjarlais R., Eisenberg L., Good B., Kleinman A. *World Mental Health: Problems and Priorities in Developing Countries*. New York: Oxford University Press; 1995.

17. Guze S. B., Robins E. L. I. 1970, Suicide and primary affective disorders, *Br. J. Psychiatry*, **117**(539): 437.

18. Wells K., Sturm R., Sherbourne C., Meredith L. *Caring for Depression: A RAND Study*. Cambridge, MA: Harvard University Press; 1996.

19. Penninx B. W. J. H., Beekman A. T. F., Honig A., et al. 2001, Depression and cardiac mortality: results from a community-based longitudinal study, *Arch. Gen. Psychiatry*, **58**(3): 221.

20. May M., McCarron P., Stansfeld S., et al. 2002, Does psychological distress predict the risk of ischemic stroke and transient ischemic attack? The Caerphilly Study, *Stroke*, **33**(1): 7.

21. Judd L. L., Martin P. P., Wells K. B., Rapaport M. H. 1996, Socioeconomic burden of subsyndromal depressive symptoms and major depression in a sample of the general population, *Am. J. Psychiatry*, **153**: 1411.

22. Sherbourne C. D., Wells K. B., Hays R. D. 1994, Subthreshold depression and depressive disorder: clinical characteristics of general medical and mental health specialty outpatients, *Am. J. Psychiatry*, **1**(51): 1.

23. APA Task Force. 1985, Tricyclic antidepressants – blood level measurements and clinical outcome: an APA Task Force report. Task Force on the Use of Laboratory Tests in Psychiatry, *Am. J. Psychiatry*, **142**(2): 155.

24. Eap C., Sirot E., Baumann P. 2004, Therapeutic monitoring of antidepressants in the era of pharmacogenetics studies, *Ther. Drug. Monit.*, **26**(2): 152.

25. Gram L., Kragh-Sorensen P., Kristensen C., Moller M., Pedersen O., Thayssen P. 1984, Plasma level monitoring of antidepressants: theoretical basis and clinical application, *Adv. Biochem. Psychopharmacol.*, **39**: 399.

26. Mann K., Hiemke C., Schmidt L., Bates D. 2006, Appropriateness of therapeutic drug monitoring for antidepressants in routine psychiatric inpatient care, *Ther. Drug. Monit.*, **28**(1): 83.

27. Kalow W. 2006, Pharmacogenetics and pharmacogenomics: origin, status, and the hope for personalized medicine, *Pharmacogenomics J.*, **6**(3): 162.

28. Malhotra A., Murphy G., Kennedy J. 2004, Pharmacogenetics of psychotropic drug response, *Am. J. Psychiatry*, **161**(5): 780.

29. Weinshilboum R., Wang L. 2004, Pharmacogenomics: bench to bedside, *Nat. Rev. Drug. Discov.*, **3**(9): 739.

30. Ingelman-Sundberg M. 2004, Pharmacogenetics of cytochrome P450 and its applications in drug therapy: the past, present and future, *Trends Pharmacol. Sci.*, **25**(4): 193.

31. Lundqvist E., Johansson I., Ingelman-Sundberg M. 1999, Genetic mechanisms for duplication and multiduplication of the human CYP2D6 gene and methods for detection of duplicated CYP2D6 genes, *Gene*, **226**(2): 327.

32. Mendoza R., Wan Y.-J., Poland R. E., et al. 2001, CYP2D6 polymorphism in a Mexican American population, *Clin. Pharmacol. Ther.*, **70**(6): 552.

33. Wan Y.-J., Poland R. E., Han G., et al. 2001, Analysis of the CYP2D6 gene polymorphism and enzyme activity in African-Americans in Southern California, *Pharmacogenetics*, **11**(6): 489.

34. Luo H.-R., Aloumanis V., Lin K.-M., Gurwitz D., Wan Y.-J. 2004, Polymorphisms of CYP2C19 and CYP2D6 in Israeli ethnic groups, *Am. J. Pharmacogenomics*, **4**(6): 395.

35. Luo H.-R., Wan Y.-J. 2006, Polymorphisms of genes encoding phase I enzymes in Mexican Americans – an ethnic comparison study, *Curr. Pharmacogenomics*, **4**(4): 345.

36. DeVane C. L. 1994, Pharmacogenetics and drug metabolism of newer antidepressant agents, *J. Clin. Psychiatry*, **55** Suppl: 38.

37. Lessard E., Yessine M. A., Hamelin B. A., O'Hara G., LeBlanc J., Turgeon J. 1999, Influence of CYP2D6 activity on the disposition and cardiovascular toxicity of the antidepressant agent venlafaxine in humans, *Pharmacogenetics*, **9**(4): 435.

38. Yin O., Wing Y., Cheung Y., et al. 2006, Phenotype–genotype relationship and clinical effects of citalopram in Chinese patients, *J. Clin. Psychopharmacol.*, **26**(4): 367.

39. Luo H.-R., Gaedigk A., Aloumanis V., Wan Y.-J. 2005, Identification of CYP2D6 impaired functional alleles in Mexican Americans, *Eur. J. Clin. Pharmacol.*, **61**(11): 797.

40. Luo H.-R., Poland R. E., Lin K.-M., Wan Y.-J. 2006, Genetic polymorphism of cytochrome P450 2C19 in Mexican Americans: a cross-ethnic comparative study, *Clin. Pharmacol. Ther.*, **80**(1): 33.

41. Harper P. A., Wong J. M. Y., Lam M. S. M., Okey A. B. 2002, Polymorphisms in the human AH receptor, *Chem. Biol. Interact.*, **141**(1–2): 161.

42. Brinkmann U., Eichelbaum M. 2001, Polymorphisms in the ABC drug transporter gene MDR1, *Pharmacogenomics J.*, **1**(1): 59.

43. Saito S., Iida A., Sekine A., et al. 2002, Three hundred twenty-six genetic variations in genes encoding nine members of ATP-binding cassette, subfamily B (ABCB/MDR/TAP), in the Japanese population, *J. Hum. Genet.*, **47**(1): 38.

44. Baumann P., Eap C. B., Muller W. E., Tillement J. P. *Alpha-Acid Glycoprotein: Genetics, Biochemistry, Physiological Functions and Pharmacology*. New York, NY: Alan R. Liss, Inc.; 1989.

45. Duché J. C., Urien S., Simon N., Malaurie E., Monnet I., Barr J. 2000, Expression of the genetic variants of human alpha-1-acid glycoprotein in cancer, *Clin. Biochem.*, **33**(3): 197.

46. Barker E. L., Blakely R. D. Norepinephrine and serotonin transporters: molecular targets of antidepressant drugs. In: F. E. Bloom and D. J. Kupfer, eds. *Psychopharmacology: The Fourth Generation of Progress*. New York, NY: Raven Press; 1995. p. 321.

47. Nelson J. C. 1999, A review of the efficacy of serotonergic and noradrenergic reuptake inhibitors for treatment of major depression, *Biol. Psychiatry*, **46**(9): 1301.

48. Schatzberg A. F., Schildkraut J. J. Recent studies on norepinephrine systems in mood disorders. In: F. E. Bloom and. D. J. Kupfer, eds. *Psychopharmacology: The Fourth Generation of Progress*. New York, NY: Raven Press; 1995. p. 911.

49. Lesch K. P., Bengel D., Heils A., et al. 1996, Association of anxiety-related traits with a polymorphism in the serotonin transporter gene regulatory region, *Science*, **274**(5292): 1527.

50. Greenberg B. D., McMahon F. J., Murphy D. L. 1998, Serotonin transporter candidate gene studies in affective disorders and personality: promises and potential pitfalls, *Mol. Psychiatry*, **3**(3): 186.

51. Hariri A. R., Mattay V. S., Tessitore A., et al. 2002, Serotonin transporter genetic variation and the response of the human amygdala, *Science*, **297**(5580): 400.

52. Yu Y. W., Tsai S. J., Chen T. J., Lin C. H., Hong C. J. 2002, Association study of the serotonin transporter promoter polymorphism and symptomatology and antidepressant response in major depressive disorders, *Mol. Psychiatry*, **7**(10): 1115.

53. Smeraldi E., Zanardi R., Benedetti F., Di Bella D., Perez J., Catalano M. 1998, Polymorphism within the promoter of the serotonin transporter gene and antidepressant efficacy of fluvoxamine, *Mol. Psychiatry*, **3**(6): 508.

54. Pollock B. G., Ferrell R. E., Mulsant B. H., et al. 2000, Allelic variation in the serotonin transporter promoter affects onset of paroxetine treatment response in late-life depression, *Neuropsychopharmacology*, **23**(5): 587.

55. Serretti A., Zanardi R., Rossini D., Cusin C., Lilli R., Smeraldi E. 2001, Influence of tryptophan hydroxylase and serotonin transporter genes on fluvoxamine antidepressant activity, *Mol. Psychiatry*, **6**(5): 586.

56. Rausch J. L., Johnson M. E., Fei Y. J., et al. 2002, Initial conditions of serotonin transporter kinetics and genotype: influence on SSRI treatment trial outcome, *Biol. Psychiatry*, **51**(9): 723.

57. Zanardi R., Serretti A., Rossini D., et al. 2001, Factors affecting fluvoxamine antidepressant activity: influence of pindolol and 5-HTTLPR in delusional and nondelusional depression, *Biol. Psychiatry*, **50**(5): 323.

58. Kim D. K., Lim S. W., Lee S., et al. 2000, Serotonin transporter gene polymorphism and antidepressant response, *Neuroreport*, **11**(1): 215.

59. Yoshida K., Ito K., Sato K., et al. 2002, Influence of the serotonin transporter gene-linked polymorphic region on the antidepressant response to fluvoxamine in Japanese depressed patients, *Prog. Neuropsychopharmacol. Biol. Psychiatry*, **26**(2): 383.

60. Durham L. K., Webb S. M., Milos P. M., Clary C. M., Seymour A. B. 2004, The serotonin transporter polymorphism, 5HTTLPR, is associated with a faster response time to sertraline in an elderly population with major depressive disorder, *Psychopharmacology*, **174**(4): 525.

61. Mundo E., Walker M., Cate T., Macciardi F., Kennedy J. L. 2001, The role of serotonin transporter protein gene in antidepressant-induced mania in bipolar disorder: preliminary findings, *Arch. Gen. Psychiatry*, **58**(6): 539.

62. Perlis R. H., Mischoulon D., Smoller J. W., et al. 2003, Serotonin transporter polymorphisms and adverse effects with fluoxetine treatment, *Biol. Psychiatry*, **54**(9): 879.

63. Konishi T., Calvillo M., Leng A.-S., Lin K.-M., Wan Y.-J. 2004, Polymorphisms of the dopamine D2 receptor, serotonin transporter, and GABAA receptor [beta]3 subunit genes and alcoholism in Mexican-Americans, *Alcohol*, **32**(1): 45.

64. Massat I., Souery D., Lipp O., et al. 2000, A European multicenter association study of HTR2A receptor polymorphism in bipolar affective disorder, *Am. J. Med. Genet.*, **96**(2): 136.

65. Serretti A., Lilli R., Lorenzi C., Smeraldi E. 1999, No association between serotonin-2A receptor gene polymorphism and psychotic symptomatology of mood disorders, *Psychiatry Res.*, **86**(3): 203.

66. Bondy B., Spaeth M., Offenbaecher M., et al. 1999, The T102C polymorphism of the 5-HT2A-receptor gene in fibromyalgia, *Neurobiol. Dis.*, **6**(5): 433.

67. Du L., Bakish D., Lapierre Y. D., Ravindran A. V., Hrdina P. D. 2000, Association of polymorphism of serotonin 2A receptor gene with suicidal ideation in major depressive disorder, *Am. J. Med. Genet.*, **96**: 56.

68. Tiihonen J., Kuikka J., Bergstrom K., et al. 1995, Altered striatal dopamine re-uptake site densities in habitually violent and non-violent alcoholics, *Nat. Med.*, **1**(7): 654.

69. Vandenbergh D. J., Persico A. M., Hawkins A. L., et al. 1992, Human dopamine transporter gene(DAT1) maps to chromosome 5p15.3 and displays a VNTR, *Genomics*, **14**(4): 1104.

70. Muramatsu T., Higuchi S. 1995, Dopamine transporter gene polymorphism and alcoholism, *Biochem. Biophys. Res. Commun.*, **211**(1): 28.

71. Parsian A., Zhang Z. H. 1997, Human dopamine transporter gene polymorphism (VNTR) and alcoholism, *Am. J. Med. Genet.*, **74**: 480.

72. Sander T., Harms H., Podschus J., et al. 1997, Allelic association of a dopamine transporter gene polymorphism in alcohol dependence with withdrawal seizures or delirium, *Biol. Psychiatry*, **41**(3): 299.

73. Inada T., Sugita T., Dobashi I., et al. 1996, Dopamine transporter gene polymorphism and psychiatric symptoms seen in schizophrenic patients at their first episode, *Am. J. Med. Genet.*, **67**: 406.

74. Barr C. L., Xu C., Kroft J., et al. 2001, Haplotype study of three polymorphisms at the dopamine transporter locus confirm linkage to attention-deficit/hyperactivity disorder, *Biol. Psychiatry*, **49**(4): 333.

75. Greenwood T. A., Alexander M., Keck P. E., et al. 2001, Evidence for linkage disequilibrium between the dopamine transporter and bipolar disorder, *Am. J. Med. Genet.*, **105**: 145.

76. Schramm N. L., McDonald M. P., Limbird L. E. 2001, The alpha(2a)-adrenergic receptor plays a protective role in mouse behavioral models of depression and anxiety, *J. Neurosci.*, **21**(13): 4875.

77. González-Maeso J., Rodríguez-Puertas R., Meana J. J., García-Sevilla J. A., Guimón J. 2002, Neurotransmitter receptor-mediated activation of G-proteins in brains of suicide victims with mood disorders: selective supersensitivity of alpha 2A-adrenoceptors, *Mol. Psychiatry*, **7**: 755.

78. Schittecatte M., Dumont F., Machowski R., et al. 2002, Mirtazapine, but not fluvoxamine, normalizes the blunted REM sleep response to clonidine in depressed patients: implications for subsensitivity of alpha2-adrenergic receptors in depression, *Psychiatry Res.*, **109**(1): 1.

79. Marazziti D., Baroni S., Masala I., et al. 2001, Correlation between platelet alpha(2)-adrenoreceptors and symptom severity in major depression, *Neuropsychobiology*, **44**(3): 122.

80. Zill P., Baghai T. C., Engel R., et al. 2003, Beta-1-adrenergic receptor gene in major depression: influence on antidepressant treatment response, *Am. J. Med. Genet.*, **120B**(1): 85.

81. Szegedi A., Rujescu D., Tadic A., et al. 2004, The catechol-O-methyltransferase Val108/158Met polymorphism affects short-term treatment response to mirtazapine, but not to paroxetine in major depression, *Pharmacogenomics J.*, **5**(1): 49.

82. Sabol S. Z., Hu S., Hamer D. 1998, A functional polymorphism in the monoamine oxidase A gene promoter, *Hum. Genet.*, **103**(3): 273.

83. Kunugi H., Ishida S., Kato T., et al. 1999, A functional polymorphism in the promoter region of monoamine oxidase-A gene and mood disorders, *Mol. Psychiatry*, **4**(4): 393.

84. Ibanez A., Perez de Castro I., Fernandez-Piqueras J., Saiz-Ruiz J. 2000, Association between the low-functional MAO-A gene promoter and pathological gambling, *Am. J. Med. Genet.*, **96**: 464.

85. Bellivier F., Leboyer M., Courtet P., et al. 1998, Association between the tryptophan hydroxylase gene and manic-depressive illness, *Arch. Gen. Psychiatry*, **55**(1): 33.

86. Nielsen D. A., Virkkunen M., Lappalainen J., et al. 1998, A tryptophan hydroxylase gene marker for suicidality and alcoholism, *Arch. Gen. Psychiatry*, **55**(7): 593.

87. Serretti A., Lorenzi C., Cusin C., et al. 2003, SSRIs antidepressant activity is influenced by Gβ3 variants, *Eur. Neuropsychopharmacol.*, **13**(2): 117.

88. Murphy G. M., Kremer C., Rodrigues H., Schatzberg A. F. 2003, The apolipoprotein E e4 allele and antidepressant efficacy in cognitively intact elderly depressed patients, *Biol. Psychiatry*, **54**(7): 665.

89. Russo-Neustadt A. A., Chen M. J. 2005, Brain-derived neurotrophic factor and antidepressant activity, *Curr. Pharm. Des.*, **11**(12): 1495.

90. Lan T., Loh E., Wu M., et al. 2008, Performance of a neuro-fuzzy model in predicting weight changes of chronic schizophrenic patients exposed to antipsychotics, *Mol. Psychiatry*, **13**(12): 1129.

91. Lin C., Wang Y., Chen J., et al. 2008, Artificial neural network prediction of clozapine response with combined pharmacogenetic and clinical data, *Comput. Methods Programs Biomed.*, **91**(2): 91.

92. Serretti A., Smeraldi E. 2004, Neural network analysis in pharmacogenetics of mood disorders, *BMC Med. Genet.*, **5**(1): 27.

93. Sproule B., Naranjo C., Türksen I. 2002, Fuzzy pharmacology: theory and applications, *Trends Pharmacol. Sci.*, **23**(9): 412.

94. Lesko L., Woodcock J. 2004, Translation of pharmacogenomics and pharmacogenetics: a regulatory perspective, *Nat. Rev. Drug. Discov.*, **3**(9): 763.

Index